Raising Healthy Children

By

Thomas Welch

2014.

Dedication

To Julie Belanger, Betty Conger and Lou Gamalski who developed many of the concepts in this book and who have shown over many years remarkable generosity of spirit, and dedication and devotion to helping at-risk children.

May your lives be full of many blessings, joy and contentment.

Index

The Goal of this Program

The purpose of this book is to provide parents and children the information they need to live and grow in healthy ways, both physically and emotionally. It is intended to provide life skills and support for all families, but especially those dealing with chemical dependency/addiction.

The lessons and supporting activities are focused on feelings, self-esteem and self worth, coping and defenses, chemical awareness, addiction, treatment and recovery, families, peer pressure and decision making, and self care. Lessons are appropriate for all children ages 6 through 18, but especially for those who have been impacted by addiction.

Interested adults and parents are also likely to find information that is helpful to you in your own lives. Parents are encouraged to work through program materials with their children, and adult involvement is necessary for younger children 6 to 12 to explain concepts. This program can also be used for several children at once, and many of the exercises are designed that way.

Standard Lesson Contents

Each lesson starts with *Goals* and *Key Messages*. The Goals are listed to orient the parent to what the lesson is intended to achieve. The Key Messages are to inform the parent what content the child is to learn during the lesson.

Each lesson also includes a list of *Activities* that are intended for you to use to bring home the Key Message concepts to your children. It is not intended that you use all the activities listed, but to pick and choose which ones you think would work best with your child. Occasionally, a particular activity once started may not seem to be working out particularly well. In that case, just stop that activity and start a different one.

In addition, a list of *Journaling* topics is included for each lesson. On the Activities sheet, a 'high value' topic is named, and in the Supplemental section that topic as well as other possibilities are listed. Parents may want to use a specific topic with the children (if one seems to be particularly relevant) or let each child pick out one from the Supplemental list that is interesting to the individual child. Journaling is a terrific skill for a child of any age to learn and practice. I believe that children who learn journaling at an early age are very likely to continue to use it as adults.

The *Seven C's* is the key concept of this entire program. That is why you will find the Seven C's chart included in every lesson. The Seven C's basically makes it clear to children that they cannot influence any aspect of addiction that may be present in their homes, but that they can take care of themselves in other ways.

Every lesson also contains a *Review* section, which allows the parents to briefly recap what was discussed during the whole lesson (or to quiz the children if such is not too stressful) and answer any questions the children may still have.

The *Serenity Pledge* ends every lesson. It is slightly but significantly different than the one widely used in 12-step programs. First it is a pledge rather than a prayer to be more accessible to those without a religious background, although you may call it the Serenity Prayer with your children if you wish. The second difference, a very important one, is that this version of Serenity focuses the child on people rather than on things, emphasizing children cannot change other people but can change themselves.

After the Serenity Pledge, which concludes the lesson, there are several *Supplemental* documents included which either support an Activity listed earlier, or (while not a formal part of the lesson) may further inform the parents (and/or children) on issues and concepts related to the main body of the lesson. These latter items can be used in the lesson or not, depending on your assessment of them.

It is recommended that no more than one lesson (of the nine in this book) is covered in a given day.

Your Role as Parents

To elicit relevant information from your children by active listening, reflecting feelings back, using open-ended questions, clarifying, making positive comments, silence, summarizing and remaining non-judgmental.

Active Listening: nodding, making eye contact, and lots of uh-huhs and mm-hmms

Reflecting Feelings Back: saying things like "It sounds like that was tough for you"

Using Open-Ended Questions: avoiding questions that can be answered with a 'yes' or 'no'; saying things like "what were you thinking then" or "how did that feel"

Clarifying: when your child makes a confusing sentence, restate it in simpler form using the child's words, not yours

Making Positive Comments: when there is appropriate opportunity to make a positive comment to your child, do so

Silence: Give your child time to think about his or her response.   Remember the time spent thinking about an answer is as important as the answer itself

Summarizing: at regular intervals, summarize a few of the main things you have been talking about

Remaining Non-Judgmental: this can be very difficult, especially with one's own children. There is always the temptation to instill rather than to learn together. But it is extremely important to remain non-judgmental so that the children are comfortable and open rather than defensive.

Parents to Children

I want to tell you a little about what we are going to be doing today.

We will talk about the unhealthy choices that some people make, for example using chemicals such as alcohol, marijuana and other drugs to make their uncomfortable feelings go away for a short while. We will talk about another unhealthy drug, tobacco, that people may use because their friends do or because they can't easily stop using it.

We will talk about what addiction is, and also discuss unhealthy relationships in which people sometimes find themselves. Addiction is also called chemical dependency in hospitals. Addiction and chemical dependency are exactly the same thing, and they mean a person is dependent on using a drug in a harmful way, just to get through the day.

We will give you true information that you can believe about the consequences of making unhealthy choices especially as concerns chemical use. We will learn and practice skills together to make you more resilient and able to take good care of yourselves.

And, we want you to have fun while you learn.

Lesson One: Feelings

<u>Goals:</u>   Children …

1. are able to identify and express both comfortable and uncomfortable feelings
2. learn that all feelings are OK and to recognize their feelings
3. understand how feelings may affect them emotionally and in their actions
4. learn how to handle their feelings in safe ways
5. learn to identify safe people with whom they can share their feelings and get support

<u>Key Messages:</u>

Everyone has feelings. In fact, everybody has all the feelings we can think of at one time or another. This means that feelings are neither good nor bad, they just are. Feelings are signals to pay attention to. They may signal us it's time to take action.

Rather than good and bad feelings, it's more helpful to think of them as comfortable and uncomfortable. While there are no wrong feelings, there are wrong ways to handle feelings. We want you to learn that there are three things we cannot do with our feelings, especially the feeling of anger - hurt ourselves, hurt others or break things.

While we work through our Healthy Children guide, you

will have many feelings about what we discuss. You may have several feelings at the same time. As your (mom/dad/grandma/grandpa, etc.) we want you to learn to share your feelings with us during this time together, and with other safe people when we're not around. Or, you can share your feelings just with yourself through journaling (which is writing down what you think about a given topic), meditation, or other techniques. We want you to learn to connect to your own feelings and to listen to the feelings of others without passing judgment.

We will discuss how "stuffing" our uncomfortable feelings usually leads to anger, depression, and frustration. And, if we turn off our feelings we don't get to choose which ones go off; in fact, we move to a state where we cannot feel anything at all.

We will learn that talking about our uncomfortable feelings makes them easier to deal with and helps us avoid making unhealthy choices. We want you to learn to accept all your feelings, even the uncomfortable ones, as gifts that connect us to the world around us.

Ice Breakers

There may be occasions when several parents follow this program together with their children. The following ice breakers can be used at the beginning of the Feelings lesson for groups of children who don't know each other well, to get everyone comfortable.

Yarn Toss - we form a circle with an adult holding a ball of yarn. The adult holds on to the end of the yarn, then calls out the name of a child across the circle and tosses the ball of yarn to that child. The child takes hold of the yarn, names another child across the circle and, while continuing to hold on to a section of the yarn, tosses the remaining yarn ball to the next child. And so it goes until everyone is holding on to a portion of the yarn, forming a giant spider web, and the remaining yarn ball is tossed back to the originating parent.

Purpose: We talk about how we are all connected, how we can accomplish things together (such as raising the web, lowering it, tightening it, and so on (note to parents, do raise the web, lower it, etc.), how sometimes people can affect us in ways we don't like or that affect us negatively such as pulling on the yarn unexpectedly or dropping it.

Name Game - We form a circle and ask for a volunteer to start. The volunteer tells us his or her name, how many brothers and sisters, and one favorite thing to do. Then we go around the circle. Each child must start with the original volunteer and repeats what the volunteer said, and what all the others coming after said, before adding his or her own information. We try to see who can remember the most, with others helping when we get stuck. At the end, we celebrate our good memories.

Purpose: to get to know each other

We talk about what our favorite time of year is, and why

Purpose: to share something pleasant

Rose and Thorn – children and parents talk in turn about something positive and something negative that has happened to them recently, and how it felt when it happened.

Purpose: to practice identifying and articulating feelings.

Activities

Feelings Rocks – Eight to ten fist-size rocks are selected to be put into a canvas bag. Each rock has had painted on it the name of an uncomfortable feeling. The first participant carries the bag around the room, preferable at arm's length, and then reports how heavy the bag is. This first child then takes a rock out of the bag without looking, reads the feeling, then says, "One time I felt ___(the feeling from the rock)___ was when _____." Children and parents continue to walk the bag, selecting a rock out of it, and discussing a time when they felt the way their particular rock dictates. The bag keeps getting lighter as the rocks are removed and the children learn that as we share our uncomfortable feelings, we reduce the load we carry around.

Note: if there isn't time to prepare the Feelings Rocks, you can do a Feelings Bag (see lesson two for instructions). Also, be prepared to explain in simple terms what the individual feelings are, for the younger children. For example, "The feeling 'envy' is what you might feel if somebody else has something that you would like to have."

Purpose: for children to learn that we can ease the burden of uncomfortable feelings just by talking about them.

Journals – each parent and child writes about an uncomfortable feeling that he or she has a lot, that's hard to tell other people about.

Purpose: children learn that it is okay to talk about uncomfortable feelings.

Tower Building with Cups – gather participants into small teams. First we build a tower with our non-dominant hand only and without communicating to our teammates. Next we try with our off-hand but we can communicate. Finally, we build a tower together with both hands, freely communicating.

Purpose: to demonstrate to the child that it's fun to cooperate and that communication makes building easier.

Scratch Art – enjoy scratching away the wax!

Purpose: to illustrate to the child that we may have to work to discover our feelings and we may have many different ones (different colors) at the same time.

(Scratch art is an 8 ½ x 11 sheet of waxy paper, showing black on top, other colors appearing when the black wax is scraped away.)

Journals - we write about an uncomfortable feeling that we have a lot, that's hard to tell other people about. At the end, we have a chance to share what we have written.

Purpose: to process our uncomfortable feelings.

Susan's Day – Each child draws a picture of Susan. A parent makes up some negative things to say about Susan's day (for example, she missed the school bus) and some positive things (she told a joke and the other kids laughed). The parent cites about the same number of negative things as positive things, for example, one negative, then two positives, then three negatives, then one positive, etc. Each child either tears off a piece of the picture (negative experience for Susan) or tapes a piece back on (positive experience for Susan). Some examples of statements that can be used are included in the Supplemental materials at the end of this lesson.

Purpose: when we finish, we understand that even though her day has been difficult, by the end of the day Susan has been "put back together" again.

Paper Wad - we write down on a slip of paper an uncomfortable feeling we have had, then another and another. Taking turns, we pick one of the slips, talk about it, then wad it up and toss it into a wastepaper basket.

Purpose: this is another way to understand that by talking about an uncomfortable feeling we can 'throw it away'.

Balloons - we write an uncomfortable feeling on a balloon with a marker. Then we blow up the balloon but do not tie it, just pinch it shut with our fingers. When everyone is done, we take turns telling what word we have written on our balloon, then let the balloon go. This activity can also be done with a paper airplane.

Purpose: we come to understand that we can "let go" of uncomfortable feelings by talking about them.

Self Portrait - we each draw a picture of ourselves and then, inside the picture or around the picture, add words or pictures denoting both comfortable and uncomfortable feelings we may sometimes have. At the end, we will have a chance to share how our picture has meaning to us.

Purpose: so the child can connect feelings to his or her person.

Feelings Charades – let all the children see the 'feelings faces' chart. Then a child volunteer (or a parent, if younger children need an example) picks a face to imitate and other children and the parents try to guess what feeling the volunteer is imitating. All the children and parents do the same in turn. If helps if you can make copies of the faces chart (see next page) and give one to each participant to help with the guessing.

Purpose: to have fun with feelings.

How are You Feeling Today?

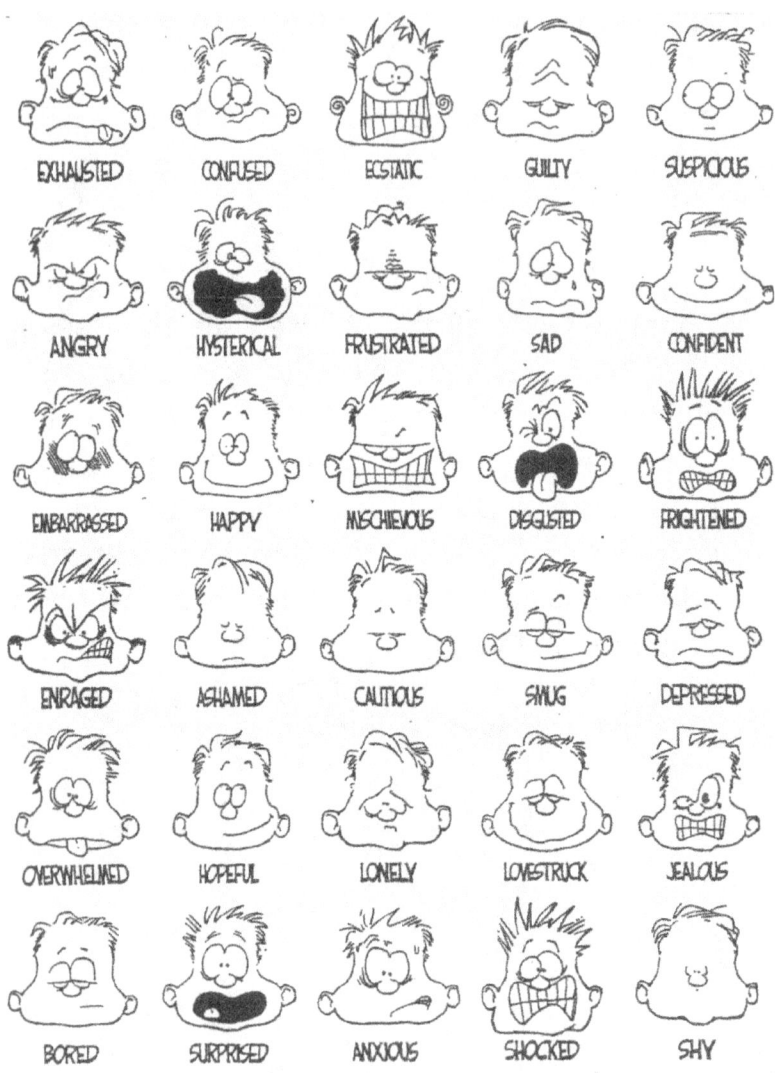

Journaling

Some suggested topics for this lesson are:

1. "An uncomfortable feeling that I have a lot, that's hard to tell other people about, is...".

2. "I'm special because..."

3. "One thing I like about myself is..."

4. "One thing I can do well is..."

5. "The most important person or thing in my life is..."

6. "What stresses me (or gets me mad) the most is..."

Often, we give the child a choice of topics. When everyone is finished (including the parent), we may share what we have written.

The Seven C's

Perhaps the most important element of this entire program is for children to learn that they are not to blame for the problems their parents may be having. This is especially true if addiction is involved. The Seven C's is important for children to practice because most children, especially younger ones, have an exaggerated sense of their central role in the family.

The Seven C's goes like this:

You didn't **C**ause it

You can't **C**ure it

You can't **C**ontrol it

But you **C**an take care of yourself, by

Making healthy **C**hoices for yourself

Communicating your feelings, and

Celebrating who you are

Check out your child's version on the next page!

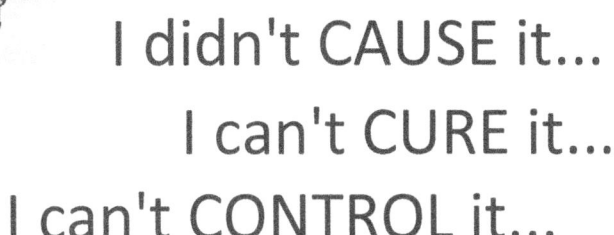

I didn't CAUSE it...

I can't CURE it...

I can't CONTROL it...

I can take CARE of myself by:

COMMUNICATING My

Feelings,

Making Healthy CHOICES and

CELEBRATING Me!

Feelings Review

Why do you think addiction is sometimes called a "feelings disease"?
Answer: because many people who abuse drugs do so to avoid or deaden uncomfortable feelings

Should people be criticized if they make us uncomfortable by expressing their feelings?
Answer: No, as long as they express themselves appropriately. We are all entitled to our feelings.

Why are there no "bad" feelings?
Answer: because everyone has all the feelings at one time or another, so we are not "good" or "bad" because of our feelings. Everyone has a right to one's feelings.

Is it better to be angry or to not feel anything?
Answer: It is healthier to be angry as long as we deal with our anger constructively, such as by talking it over with someone we trust, by journaling, exercising, and so on.

What are three things we should not do when we are angry or have another uncomfortable feeling?
Answer: hurt ourselves, hurt others or break things. *If someone answers "do drugs", say "that's right, because we would be hurting ourselves."*

What was the message of the 'Feelings Rocks'?
Answer: that uncomfortable feelings can be a load to carry, but talking about these feelings helps us release them and lighten our load

Do people sometimes have more than one feeling at a time? *Answer*, yes

Describe a situation where you might have 'mixed feelings'.
Answer: One example - your best friend got accepted into her first choice college and you also applied there but did not get accepted. You might be happy for her and also jealous.

If a chemically dependent (addicted) person is using, what are some of the feelings his/her family members might have?
Answer: fear, anger, frustration, exasperation, depression, and more

Homework Assignment

When you brush your teeth before going to bed tonight, look at yourself in the mirror and tell yourself, **"I am OK!"**

OR

Look into a mirror and say "I am a loving person … I am special" and think about why you are special.

What I Liked Best About Today

Ask your child,

What did you like best about today?

Did you enjoy the time we spent together?

What is one important thing you learned today that you

didn't know before?

Serenity Pledge

Grant me the <u>Serenity</u> to accept the

people I cannot change,

The <u>Courage</u> to change the person I can,

And the <u>Wisdom</u> to know that person is me.

- This ends today's lesson on Feelings!

Recommended Video

Twee Fiddle and Huff

Author: Remboldt
Publication Date: 30-Sep-1998
Publisher: Hazelden Professional

This video is a cartoon with three main characters who learn that they have a lot in common. They get help from a kind teacher who includes them in a regular group where other children share their sadness about a parent's addiction.

Susan's Day

Here are some examples of statements that can be used for this activity.

- Susan's best friend told her she had to move to a different city
- Susan's friend's family asked if she could go on a short trip with them
- Susan's bike was not where she left it before school
- It's Susan's turn to clean the house or mow the lawn
- Susan is going to stay at her grandma's for 2 weeks
- A friend told Susan a secret that Susan feels an adult should hear
- Susan just found out she is going swimming with a friend
- Susan just found out she is going to summer school
- Susan just heard that she has the same teacher next fall as her best friend
- One of Susan's parents gave her a big hug
- Susan just found $10 on the sidewalk
- One of Susan's brothers or sisters just made a big mistake and her folks blamed it on her
- Susan just ate a whole pizza by herself
- Susan just called someone by the wrong name

Parent to Child, Anger Management Techniques

<u>Talk it out</u>:   If someone makes you angry you can talk to that person about it, or to a responsible adult.

<u>Take 5 deep breaths</u>:   Taking very deep breaths and relaxing your muscles will help you calm down very quickly. When you are calm, you can act with a clear head.

<u>Take your anger out on an object that won't be hurt</u>: Sometimes people hit pillows when they are angry because it doesn't hurt them or the pillow. Never hit something that could be broken or that would hurt you if you hit it.

<u>Play a sport</u>:   Physical activities may help many people express some of their anger, energy and frustration in a positive way.

<u>Turn on some music</u>:   Music is a powerful way of changing your mood.

<u>Think about a peaceful place</u>:   Many people use their imagination to help calm down or relax. They imagine that they are swimming in the ocean or flying through the clouds or relaxing in a safe place.

<u>Make a lot of noise in a place where you won't bother</u>

anyone: Making noise sometimes helps get your anger out, but you have to do it in a place where, and at a time when you won't bother anyone.

Count to 10:   Holding your temper and gaining self-control is important for all of us.

Get some advice: If you find yourself getting angry about something over and over again, you may need some advice from an adult you trust.

For Children, Healthy Ways to Handle Anger

Tell someone you're angry.
Talk to yourself in the mirror about your anger.
Hit a pillow.
Jump up and down.
Cry.
Hit the floor with a rolled-up newspaper.
Smash play dough or clay.
Hit a bed with your fist, and yell, "I'M SO ANGRY!!!"

Tear and crumple up newspapers, magazines, or old phone books and fill a garbage bag.

Go into a safe room to get some "space".

Control your breathing; take several slow, deep breaths, breathing in through your nose and out through your mouth.

Walk away.

Try exercising: take a walk, ride a bike, run or jog, do yoga, boxing, karate or judo; go swimming and hit the water.

Count to 10 very slowly.

Lie on a bed with your feet in the air. Kick your feet back and forth and yell, "AHHHHH!" or "I'M ANGRY!!!"

Take a small towel and use it to hit a couch, chair or
bed while saying, "I'm so angry!"

Play an angry song on a musical instrument; sing an angry
song.

Beat a drum.

Do an angry dance.

Go to a playground; bounce or kick a ball. Swing.

Go to a pond, lake, river or ocean; throw rocks into the
water.

Write the whole story down.

Start a project.

For Parents, Dealing with Painful Feelings

Feelings of hurt or anger can be some of the most difficult to face. We can feel so vulnerable, frightened, and powerless when these feelings appear. And these feelings may trigger memories of other times when we felt powerless.

Sometimes, to gain a sense of control, we may punish the people around us, whether they are people we blame for these feelings or innocent bystanders. We may try to "get even," or we may manipulate behind people's backs to gain a sense of power over the situation.

These actions may give us a temporary feeling of satisfaction, but they only postpone facing our pain. Feeling hurt does not have to be so frightening. We do not have to work so hard to avoid it.

Sometimes we may be angry because we have drawn a hard consequence as a result of an inappropriate action of our own.

While hurt feelings aren't much fun, they are still just feelings.

We can surrender to them, feel them, and go on. Emotional pain does not have to devastate us. We can sit still, feel the pain, figure out if there's something we need to do to take care of ourselves, and then set the feeling aside and go on with our lives.

We don't have to act in haste; we do not have to punish others to get control over our feelings. We can begin by sharing our hurt feelings with others. This brings relief and often healing to them and us.

Eventually, we learn the lesson that real power comes from allowing ourselves to be vulnerable enough to feel hurt. Real power comes from knowing we can take care of ourselves, even when we feel emotional pain. Real power comes when we stop holding others responsible for our pain and take responsibility for all our feelings.

Sometimes people are angry for good reasons. If we are angry because someone has hurt us, that is understandable. Every person has certain rights that should not be taken away. We must learn to stick up for ourselves and our rights in a constructive way.

Today, I will surrender to my feelings, even the emotionally painful ones. Instead of acting in haste, or striking out to punish someone, I will stay in the moment and be vulnerable enough to feel in full, and share my hurt when I am able.

For the Child,

What to Do When I'm Depressed, Bored or Lonely

Listen to music,   dance,   play computer games,   do something with my family,   play a board game,   play basketball/football/baseball,   go fishing,   go boating, go skiing,   see a friend,   make a new friend,   play an instrument,   go skateboarding,   go biking,   go ice-skating or rollerblading,   draw or paint,   write,   read, play with a pet,   help someone,   go to the playground, go rock climbing

Go out to eat,   knit ,   crochet,   needlepoint,   cross-stitch,   rug hooking,   fashion,   give myself a manicure, pedicure, facial, hair treatment,   do homework,   start a project,   pray or meditate,   take a walk,   go for a hike, go swimming,   do arts and crafts,   go bowling,   sing, go to the sauna or Jacuzzi,   go horseback riding, garden,   go sight-seeing,   make up some comedy, play soccer,   yoga

Decorate my space,   learn something,   jump on a trampoline,   go shopping,   cook or bake,   go scuba diving or snorkeling,   go on a roller coaster,   go to the water slides,   visit someone,   write a letter,   go water skiing,   go camping,   play a card game,   go jogging, go on a picnic,   stargaze,   call someone,   sew,   do woodworking,   go hunting,   take some pictures

For Parents and Children - How to Love Yourself

<u>Stop all Criticism</u>: Criticism never changes a thing. Refuse to criticize yourself. Accept yourself exactly as you are. Everybody changes. When you criticize yourself, your changes will be negative. When you approve of yourself, your changes will be positive.

<u>Don't Scare Yourself</u>: Don't imagine some terrible thing happening. Stay in the now; stick with what is real. Find a mental image that gives you pleasure or makes you feel secure (such as meeting with your closest friends), and immediately switch your scary thoughts to a 'pleasure' thought.

<u>Be Gentle and Kind and Patient</u>: Be gentle with yourself. Be kind to yourself. Treat yourself as if you were someone you really loved.

<u>Be Kind to Your Mind</u>: Self-hatred is only hating your thoughts. Don't hate yourself for having thoughts. Gently change your thoughts in a positive direction. Beating yourself up doesn't work - try kindness!

<u>Praise Yourself</u>: Criticism breaks down the inner spirit. Praise builds it up. Praise yourself often. Tell yourself how well you are doing with every little thing. Remember, recovering one's health is a process that results in progress, not perfection.

<u>Support Yourself</u>: Find ways to support yourself

emotionally. Reach out to friends and allow them to help you. It is being strong to ask for help when you need it.

Be Loving to Your Negatives: Acknowledge that you created them to fulfill a need. Now you are finding new, positive ways to fulfill those needs. So lovingly release the old negative patterns.

Take Care Of Your Body: Learn about nutrition. What kind of fuel does your body need to have optimum energy and vitality? Find some kind of exercise that you can enjoy. Cherish and revere the temple in which you live!

Mirror Work: Look into your own eyes often. Express this growing sense of love you have for yourself. Forgive yourself. Talk to your parents, children, relatives and co-workers while looking into the mirror. Forgive them, too. At least once a day say, "*I love you and I am going to take care of you*."

Do it Now: Don't wait until you are somehow more together, or until you lose weight, or find the right person to love you, or find the right job. Begin now by doing the best you can.

Child's Worksheet - Safe People and Safe Places

My favorite place to go when I want to be alone or to think is

A place that feels good and safe to me is

If I have a problem that I don't know how to solve alone, there are people and places I can turn to for help. I could go to

A relative, friend, or neighbor I could call if I ever needed help is

This person's telephone number is

Someone I can trust and share my feelings with is

Guided Meditation to a Safe Place

This is a tool to help us calm down, or remove ourselves from a difficult situation. This activity helps children learn to go to a safe place in their minds.

Ask the children to make themselves comfortable (lying on the floor, or seated with head down, resting on arms) and relax. Ask them to take a few deep breaths and close their eyes.

Say: "Now imagine a place where you feel safe and happy and where you have everything that you want and need . . . Take yourself there . . . If you want to, take someone with you . . . Try to experience the place as fully as you can. . . Use all of your senses. . . Move around in the place . . . Touch things . . . If there are any things which you want to change, adjust them to your liking . . . Now slowly open your eyes and come back to our room and make contact with it . . . Look around, touch a few things, do whatever gets you back to our surroundings. Do you notice anything different in your present surroundings? . . . . . . Now go back to your place. . . This time notice whether you go back to the same place . . . Did you find your way easily? Do you notice anything different? . . . Stay there for a while and then open your eyes and come back here . . . Shuttle back and forth between your present surroundings and your special place so that you can learn how to get there easily . . . Now come back and stretch your arms and open your eyes.

Ask the children how they feel, compared to before. Prompt if necessary - Are you more relaxed? Do you feel refreshed? What else? Who wants to go first?

For the Child
My Birthday is Special to Me!

Sometimes it feels uncomfortable to tell others what we want or need; perhaps it makes us feel selfish. However, if we don't tell others what we want, we may never get what we need in life. We can't just hope that others will read our minds, or that they will be able to tell what we want by the hints we give them.

Part of taking care of ourselves is telling others what we like and want and also what we need. We don't always get these things. But if no one knows, it's pretty certain that we won't receive them.

When it's a couple of weeks before your birthday, fill in the blanks below. Share this with your loved ones so they know what you'd like to have happen on your special day. Most people like to recognize and please their loved ones on special days, so this list will help them know you better.

My birthday is:

The date we will celebrate my birthday is:

Menu
On my birthday what I would like for breakfast is:
On my birthday what I would like for lunch is:
On my birthday what I would like for dinner is:
On my birthday I would like this for my special dessert:

Gifts of the Heart

I know that I cannot always have what I want for my birthday. Sometimes we can't afford what I really want; sometimes I might just want too much. But it's OK to have wishes! Here are some ideas for gifts I would like that don't have to cost any money:

One impossible thing I wish for is:

I would really like it if someone would do this chore for me on my birthday:

Just for one day, I wish our family could:

If it is possible, I would really like to celebrate my birthday with the following family members:

and the following friends:

Lesson Two: Self-Esteem and Self-Worth

<u>Goals:</u>   Children learn ...

1. that everyone has special qualities, both strengths and weaknesses
2. to appreciate their capabilities and self-worth
3. it is okay to feel good about themselves
4. they cannot change what is around them when they are small
5. they can always change the way they relate to the world

<u>Key Messages:</u>

We all have special qualities (strengths and weaknesses). We all contribute to our families and communities in many positive ways. It's okay for us to feel good about ourselves. We are all lovable and capable, and *we all deserve to have a good life*.

The way others treat us sometimes affects the way we feel about ourselves. Often parents focus on the things we do wrong rather than the positives in our lives. When they do this, they do not mean to demean us. They may just be tired, or scared for us. However, what we hear from others sometimes turns into a "tape" that we learn to play back in our minds. When the "tape" we run is saying hurtful things, we need to say to ourselves, "No, that's not true. I really am ..." (the opposite of what the tape said).

While we do not always have the power to change the world around us, we can always change the way we relate to the world. In the end, changing how we relate to the world *is more important than anything else* to our happiness.

Activities

Feelings Bag – a number of slips of paper are prepared, each with a comfortable or an uncomfortable open-ended feeling statement written on it. Then the slips are put into a bag and each child and adult in turn pulls out a slip, reads the feeling inscribed there, and says "One time I felt _____ was when_____."

Examples of slips that can be put into the Feelings Bag are listed in the Supplemental materials section at the end of this lesson. You may want to underline the feelings words on the slips of paper you put into the Feelings Bag if the children are small. If not underlined, you can ask each child to first determine which is the feeling word before completing the sentence.

The 'Feelings Bag' activity is done at the start of every lesson beginning with Lesson Two (Lesson One, if 'Feelings Rocks' were not available).

Purpose: to reinforce how important handling feelings is for a healthy life.

Journals – children write about a way in which each contributes to his or her family.

Purpose: children learn they are important members of their families.

Pleasant/Painful – a piece of paper with 'pleasant' is placed in one part of the room and another with 'painful' is placed a little ways away. Then the parent reads statements and the children run to the paper that reflects how they would feel if the statement were true. In larger groups, the children learn that not everyone feels the same way for some of the statements. Some sample statements for use in this exercise are listed in the Supplemental materials section at the end of this lesson.

Purpose: children learn that what goes on around them has an effect on them, even when not directed toward any child in particular. It should be pointed out that many things are not in the child's control.

Car Wash – (for larger groups) we stand in two rows. One of us walks slowly between the rows. The rest of us simulate a "washing" motion while saying positive things to the person who is walking. We find nice things to say about the child's character (how the child acts) or complement the child's looks or style. Everyone will get the chance to walk between the rows.

Purpose: children learn how hearing even the most mundane nice things said about themselves still has a powerful positive effect on their self-esteem.

Self-esteem Hat - we use fabric markers to decorate an old hat with affirmations that are meaningful to us, using symbols or pictures to represent specific affirmations (e.g., a sun for a positive disposition). Some examples of affirmations that can be used in this exercise are listed in the Supplemental materials section at the end of this lesson.

Purpose: the child learns that being positive makes for more fun and energy.

Positive/Negative Affirmations Chart - we make a list on two poster boards of nice things we would like to hear people say about us and on the second board, negative things we would definitely not like to hear. We ask for a child to volunteer to listen while we say all the positive things. We then ask the volunteer how it felt to hear all these nice things. Then we ask the children to imagine how it would feel to hear all the negative things read. Of course, we do not read off the negative things unless two adults are present, one reading the negatives off to the other. In this case we then ask the children how it felt to hear adults say negative things to one another.

Purpose: that the child learns negative words are very painful to hear, even when they are directed toward others.

"I" and "You" Messages – Background: uncomfortable feelings that remain unexpressed never die. They are buried alive and come forth later in unexpected ways. You've got to share these feelings or they'll eat your heart out. If you take the time to really hear what others are saying, your chances of being listened to are very good. When giving feedback to others, send "I" messages instead of "You" messages. In other words, express your feelings in the first person.

For example, a parent can say, "*I'm* concerned that you have a temper problem" or a child can say "*I* feel taken for granted and unappreciated when you say I never do anything to help around here." Messages with "You" are more threatening because they sound as if you are labeling the person rather than describing the child's action: "**You** have a terrible temper" or "**You** don't appreciate anything!" Some examples of "I" versus "You" messages that can be used in this exercise are listed in the Supplemental materials section at the end of this lesson.

Purpose: to allow the child to see that accusatory statements just make a person feel attacked or threatened and usually prevent meaningful discussions.

Affirmations: children are given a piece of colored paper and color markers to make an Affirmation poster. In case some children need prompting, a few examples of children's affirmations are listed in the Supplemental materials section at the end of this lesson.

Purpose: to teach children that words have power.

Back-to-Back – participants sit back-to-back. First, one child draws a simple picture then describes it to the person sitting at his or her back. That person tries to duplicate the drawing via the original drawer's description.

Purpose: to realize that we believe others understand us better than they usually do, and to have fun.

Journaling

Some suggested topics for this lesson are:

1. "One way I contribute to my family is ...".

2. "Some ways I can influence what happens to me

   are ..."

3. "One thing I am really good at is ..."

4. "My personal hero is ..." (and why)

Often, we give the children a choice of topics. When everyone is finished (including the parent), we may share what we have written.

Self-Esteem and Self-Worth Review

What is self-esteem?
Answer: how we feel about ourselves

Can self-esteem be positive for one person and negative for another?
Answer: yes

How does negative self-esteem hold a person back?
Answer: such a person may not try new things, such a person may often feel depressed or socially isolated, such a person may try drugs because of social isolation or depression

Do we get our feelings of self-esteem and self-worth from our parents?
Answer: yes, and from other people who are important in our lives

Can we change the way we feel about ourselves?
Answer: yes

How can we start to feel more positive about ourselves?
Answer: we can stop hanging around people who put us down, and when we have a 'negative' thought we can say to ourselves, "No, that's not true. I'm really ..." (the opposite)

Do we have the power to change the world around us?
Answer: to some extent but our power can be limited by our circumstances

Do we have the power to change the way we relate to the world?

Answer: Always! And we start by changing the way we relate to the people around us

Are we really capable of accomplishing much more than we think we can?

Answer: Yes, and discovering new talent and developing new strengths brings joy to our lives!

If you could give yourself one present, what would it be?

Answer: (go around the room...) One answer might be, to be loved, appreciated and accepted just as I am

Homework Assignment

When you get up tomorrow morning, look at yourself in the mirror and tell yourself,

"I am a loving person, I am very special, and I am capable of great things"

... and think about some great things you would like to accomplish.

The Seven C's

The Seven C's goes like this:

You didn't **C**ause it

You can't **C**ure it

You can't **C**ontrol it

But you **C**an take care of yourself, by

Making healthy **C**hoices for yourself

Communicating your feelings, and

Celebrating who you are

What I Liked Best About Today

Ask your child,

What did you like best about today?

Did you enjoy the time we spent together?

What is one important thing you learned today that you

 didn't know before?

Serenity Pledge

Grant me the <u>Serenity</u> to accept the

people I cannot change,

The <u>Courage</u> to change the person I can,

And the <u>Wisdom</u> to know that person is me.

- This ends today's lesson on Self-
Esteem and Self-Worth!

Feelings Bag

Here are some examples of slips to put into the Feelings Bag:

- I felt <u>jealous</u> one time when …
- One thing that really gets me <u>mad</u> is …
- I feel <u>nervous</u> when …
- I was really <u>excited</u> one time when …
- I felt really <u>misunderstood</u> once when …
- I almost always feel <u>happy</u> when …
- I usually feel <u>depressed</u> when …
- I feel <u>thankful</u> when …
- I usually feel <u>afraid</u> when …
- I feel <u>hopeful</u> when …
- I feel <u>loving</u> when …
- I was once really <u>scared</u> when …
- Sometimes I feel <u>discouraged</u> when …
- I feel really <u>depressed</u> when I think about …
- The times I feel most <u>bored</u> are …
- I really feel <u>disgusted</u> when …
- Sometimes I just <u>don't care</u> when … (indifference)

- One time a felt really <u>proud</u> of myself was when …

- I felt really <u>disappointed</u> once when …

- I was feeling really <u>lonely</u> once when …

- Once I felt really <u>confused</u> when …

- One time I felt really <u>guilty</u> was when …

- Once I felt <u>hysterical</u> when …

- I really feel <u>confident</u> when …

- Once I felt really <u>embarrassed</u> when …

- I feel really <u>shy</u> around …

- I was <u>shocked</u> to find out that …

- One time I was very <u>disappointed</u> with a friend when …

- One thing that really <u>surprised</u> me was …

- I really feel <u>frustrated</u> when …

- I felt really <u>mischievous</u> once when I …

- I felt really <u>smug</u> once when …

- I am really <u>curious</u> about …

- I get really <u>enthusiastic</u> when …

- I get really <u>creative</u> when …

- One time I felt really <u>awed</u> was …

Pleasant / Painful

Here are some sample statements:

- We are going to grandma's house for Thanksgiving dinner
- I failed an important English test
- My mom is going to pick me up from my friend's house
- My brother will be coming to my birthday party
- My dad hit my mom last night
- I can't find my necklace
- My dad will be home when I get home from school
- I got caught stealing from the mall yesterday
- I got the best grade in the class on the test
- I saw the biggest kid in my neighborhood today when I was shooting hoops
- I will be the only one home tonight at my house
- One of my family members got arrested last night
- My mother read my journal
- I have a big event tomorrow that I have been preparing for

- My mom told me I can't tell anyone what happens at our house
- I saw my two best friends riding by in a car yesterday
- I'm going to meet my uncle at the park
- My parents are getting a divorce
- My sister is in treatment at a rehabilitation center
- My mom is having another baby soon
- My little brother took money from my bedroom
- My mom got in a loud screaming match with the neighbor
- I accidentally wet my bed
- I saw my mom at the coffee shop with someone I didn't know
- My grandparents, aunts, uncles and cousins will be coming to spend a week at our house on vacation

Self-Esteem Hat

Here are some examples of slogans for the Self-Esteem hat:

- All my feelings are OK!
- Believe! Achieve!
- I can change myself; others I can only love!
- "NO" is a complete sentence
- Think, Don't Drink!
- Stay Happy! Stay Free!
- No Hope with Dope!
- Choose Life!
- Hugs, not Drugs!
- All Families are Special!
- Tone of Voice is a Choice!
- Stress Relief is Simple - Breathe to Relieve!
- Blow Bubbles not Smoke!
- I Can Celebrate ME!
- I can say NO!

"I" versus "You" Messages

Ask the children which statement in each couplet makes them feel better about what's being said:

- "I don't understand why someone would try to hurt another person's feelings" versus "You always try to hurt people's feelings"
- "You never settle down to study on time" versus "I feel discouraged when I realize how little studying we've gotten done this week"
- "I feel annoyed when I see you use my tablet without asking" versus "You're selfish and inconsiderate of others people's property"
- "You don't listen to me when I talk to you" versus "I feel upset when people aren't polite enough to listen to me"
- "I'd really appreciate it if you'd help me with the yard work" versus "You never remember you're supposed to help with the yard work"

Affirmations

- I use put-ups only   (*to parents – we mean as opposed to 'put-downs'*)
- I tell the truth
- I am a good friend
- I can have fun
- I can ask for help
- I am a hard worker
- I always do my best
- I like to please mom and dad
- I respect myself and others
- I communicate my feelings respectfully
- I keep my body clean
- I have safe friends
- I respect my spiritual side
- I learn new things
- My work is done on time
- I exercise my mind and body
- I am unique, no one else is exactly like me
- I am an important part of my family
- I am fun to be around

Serenity Worksheet

Grant me the serenity to accept the things I cannot change

Here are some things I cannot change (in others);

1.

2.

3.

4.

5.

Courage to change the things I can

Here are some things I can change

(about me).'

1.

2.

3.

4.

5.

And the wisdom to know the difference

Here is a plan to take good care of me

1.

2.

3.

4.

5.

Shame and Guilt

Guilt is believing what we <u>did</u> is not OK.

Shame is believing who we <u>are</u> is not OK.

Shame hurts. It has its roots in the past, often in our childhoods. It focuses us backwards. Shame can stop us from taking care of ourselves in the 'now' and moving forward with our lives.

Self-Respect and Self-Esteem

Self-Respect: I take good care of myself by making healthy choices, communicating my feelings and celebrating who I am.

Self-Esteem: I feel good about myself because I know I am lovable and capable of loving others.

Cicero Quotations

ABATES DIVIDING DOUBLING FRIENDSHIP GRIEF HAPPINESS JOY MISERY

"_____ improves _____ and _____ _____ , by the _____ of our _____ and the _____ of our _____."

DILIGENT FARMER FRUIT HIMSELF NEVER PLANTS SEE TREES

"The _____ _____ _____ _____ of which he _____ will _____ _____ the _____."

answers:

"Friendship improves happiness and abates misery, by the doubling of our joy and the dividing of our grief."

"The diligent farmer plants trees of which he himself will never see the fruit."

Lesson Three: Coping and Defenses

<u>Objectives:</u>   Children learn ...

1. that everyone has problems to deal with
2. to cope with problems, which involves learning to STOP and THINK before acting
3. various problem solving skills
4. that what has worked for a child at an earlier stage of life will not necessarily work when the child is older
5. that defenses are masks that hide feelings
6. that defenses may be safe or unsafe
7. that we may *choose* to use a particular defense, or not to

<u>Key Messages:</u>

Everyone has problems. *Coping* means getting through a difficult time. There are healthy and unhealthy ways to cope. Some healthy ways are talking things over with a safe person, journaling, exercising, punching a pillow, etc. To "stuff" our feelings so that we can avoid pain is unhealthy. When we do this, eventually the dam will break and we will explode in anger. It's also unhealthy to always let another person have his way at the expense of our own interests or to hurt ourselves by stealing, overeating, gambling, meaningless sex, etc. And finally, a *very unhealthy* way to cope is to use drugs to deaden our feelings.

Defenses are ways people or animals hide or protect themselves. Animals, for example, use camouflage, playing dead, bad smells, poison, quills, hard shells, and so on to protect themselves. Animal defenses are almost always helpful because natural selection eliminates animals that use less effective defenses.

People also use defenses to hide their true feelings. Our defenses are neither good nor bad. They can be more effective or less effective. They may be safe or unsafe. Some defenses are helpful. For example, if we are around someone who is extremely irritating, we can leave or be tactful. If the person is physically aggressive we may run away, call 911, or yell out for help. In other words, a healthy defense *is one we choose*, that *keeps us safe* and is *appropriate to a situation*. If a defense keeps us from dealing with our true feelings, from facing truth and reality, then it is not healthy.

Sometimes defenses we use as *children* are less useful when we become *adults*. For example, in a home where there is substance abuse it might be very useful for a child to obey or at least not confront a parent who is abusing drugs. As an adult, however, we may choose to confront the drug use or to leave an unhealthy relationship. If, as an adult, we remain non-confrontational to the drug use of someone we care about, we can fall into an unhealthy condition known as "codependency" or "enabling" (these are the same thing). This means that we try to fix all the problems caused by another person's drug abuse and lose sight of taking care of our own needs.

As a guide, if a defense we are using *keeps us from dealing with a real problem or with our true feelings*, that defense is probably unhealthy.

Include in your discussion with your children the importance of protecting themselves by staying out of family fights or other fights, and to get help for emotional, physical or sexual abuse. Your children should also understand that if someone threatens harm, they should find an adult to tell. _Encourage them, if the first person does not help, to find another_. Talk about the right kinds of adults to tell, such as yourself, a teacher, a school counselor, etc.

Activities

Feelings Bag – as described in Lesson Two (recommended for each lesson)

Purpose: for children to learn that we can ease the burden of uncomfortable feelings just by talking about them.

Name that Defense – the children and the parents each draw a picture of an animal that uses a defense. Each then explains what the animal is, what defense it uses, and whether the defense works. Each talks about whether he or she use uses the particular defense that the drawn animal uses, and when, and does it work. Afterward, the younger children can color in the picture.

Purpose: children learn that defenses are useful, for animals and, by extension, people.

Hat Decoration - We decorate a hat (or use a hat that we decorated previously) and talk about how hats protect us from the sun and weather. We also discuss how our clothing choices, haircuts, makeup decisions and so on might be ways to hide our feelings or hide who we really are.

Purpose: to use an everyday item to think about defenses.

Leave that Coping Behind – children are asked to think of some coping mechanisms that small children often use that work when one is small but don't work as well as one gets older. (Some examples are crying, hiding under a bed, freezing when scared, and so on).

Purpose: children learn that coping strategies must be kept updated so they continue to work for us.

Mask Decoration – We make a mask out of a paper plate, using colored markers. The mask is to show a feeling, such as happiness, fear, anger, etc. Then we explain how the mask may be hiding other feelings as well, and what those other feelings might be. Children are asked whether hiding our feelings is sometimes helpful and when that might be. For example, it might be better to hide anger when dealing with overwrought adult, or to hide irritation when dealing with a difficult boss at work.

Purpose: children learn that defenses work for us just as they do for animals, as long as we use them at appropriate times and not always.

Journal - children write about a defense, either healthy or unhealthy, that they often use and then present it to the group. Parents do the same.

Purpose: children use another tool (written language) to process thinking.

Scratch Art - the black sheet represents a defense and the colors underneath represent our true feelings and the beauty of the person we are inside.

Purpose: children learn that we all have many layers to our personalities, and that we reveal more of our true selves to those closest to us.

Egg Drop – each parent teams up with a child to create a 'defense' for an egg drop. If there are insufficient parents, the some parents support more than one child. If the egg you use is fresh make sure you do the drop outside or somewhere easy to clean up. The child takes the lead in designing and building the egg 'defender' with a parent in the supporting role. Start with 5 feet of masking tape, 20 or so straws and one egg. Parent and child communicate with each other to plan a method of protecting the egg with the straws and tape. The drop is by the child, standing on a chair or bench. Success is when a raw egg doesn't break spilling yolk or a hard-boiled egg survives the drop without cracking its shell.

Purpose: children relate the activity to the defenses that we use and how we can 'crack' when the defense doesn't work.

Journaling

Some suggested topics for this lesson are:

- "The defense I use most often is …"
- Write about something that stresses you and what you do to cover up that feeling
- Write about what causes you stress and what helps reduce it
- Write about a true feeling that you cover up, and why, and do you need to?
- What would people think of you if they knew the real you?
- Make a list of healthy ways you currently cope or plan to cope

Often, we give children a choice of topics. When everyone is finished (including the parents), we may share what we have written.

Defenses Review

What are defenses?

Answer:

- means and methods of protecting ourselves from hurt or harm
- ways to avoid or resist attack
- ways we hide our true feelings to keep us safe
- ways we hide our true feelings and not deal with them at all

What are some defenses that animals and plants use for protection?

Answer:

- porcupines and cactus use quills, spines or barbs
- armadillos and turtles use shells
- chameleons use camouflage
- cheetahs, deer and rabbits use quickness
- skunks use a foul odor
- squid and octopuses use ink to hide
- snakes use fangs and sometimes poison

What are some defenses people use to hide their true feelings?

Answer:

- fighting
- crying
- rebelling
- arguing

- rationalizing or intellectualizing
- eating too much
- sleeping too much
- talking too much
- withdrawing
- stealing
- using alcohol or other drugs
- lying
- smiling
- trying to be perfect
- clowning
- anger

Do people have lots of ways to hide their true feelings?
Answer: yes

Do people sometimes hide their true feelings from themselves?
Answer: yes

What is it called when people hide their true feelings from themselves?
Answer: 'stuffing' their feelings

What generally happens when people stuff their feelings for a long time?
Answer:

- they explode in anger, or
- they get very depressed

Not all defenses are unhealthy. Some help us deal with difficult situations and protect us. But some defenses are not healthy ways to deal with our feelings. How can we tell if a defense is helpful or harmful?

Answer: if our defense keeps us from dealing with our true feelings, then it is probably not healthy.

What are some defenses that will definitely do us more harm than good?

Answer: using alcohol or other drugs to dull our feelings or engaging in illegal or self-destructive behaviors are definitely not healthy.

A common defense people use is blaming. Who would like to tell us about a time when you blamed someone else to get yourself out of trouble or so you didn't have to be punished alongside? Who would like to tell us about a time when someone else blamed you unfairly?

Sometimes when we are really angry we don't deal with it well. We fight or slap, scream obscenities, break or destroy things, hurt ourselves or just hide away and cry. We might be tempted to use alcohol or other drugs to help us forget about these painful feelings. What are some healthy alternatives to cope with uncomfortable feelings?

Answer:

- talk to someone we trust
- go for a long walk
- breathe deeply

- count slowly to ten
- meditate
- pray
- hit a pillow
- go for a bike ride
- play basketball
- take a long bath
- call a friend
- get a massage
- write in a journal
- read a list of self-affirmations
  ... and many more

Coping Review

What does 'coping' mean?
Answer: getting through a difficult time

Are there *healthy* ways of coping? What are some?
Answer:

- talking things over with a safe person,
- journaling
- exercise
- punching a pillow
- asking for help
- making a plan and carrying it out
- not hanging around people who put us down
- walking away, or if necessary, running away
- if necessary, yelling for help

What are some *unhealthy* ways people cope? Name some.
Answer:

- 'stuffing' their feelings
- stop trying and become totally passive
- isolating themselves away from other people
- eating too much or too little
- hurting themselves (such as cutting themselves, punching a wall, taking alcohol or other drugs to numb their feelings, etc.)
- risky behavior (such as unprotected sex, riding in a car with a driver under the influence, etc.)
- hurting other people (hitting, put-downs, gossip, teasing, sarcasm, being mean, etc.)

- breaking things

What do we gain by coping successfully with a difficult situation?

Answer:

- We learn how to ask for help
- We develop new strengths and capabilities
- We gain experience
- We gain personal satisfaction and feelings of confidence and control

Does everyone spend every day coping?
Answer: yes, that's called living!

Homework Assignment

Think of defenses you have been using, and see if there is one that isn't working very well for you anymore. Decide whether you can let this defense down, that is, stop using it.

OR

For a whole day, notice what defenses you use and when you use them.

OR

Try to communicate a real feeling to someone you trust and try not to use a defense.

The Seven C's

The Seven C's goes like this:

You didn't **C**ause it

You can't **C**ure it

You can't **C**ontrol it

But you **C**an take care of yourself, by

Making healthy **C**hoices for yourself

Communicating your feelings, and

Celebrating who you are

What I Liked Best About Today

Ask your child,

What did you like best about today?

Did you enjoy the time we spent together?

What is one important thing you learned today that you

didn't know before?

Serenity Pledge

Grant me the Serenity to accept the

people I cannot change,

The Courage to change the person I can,

And the Wisdom to know that person is me.

- This ends today's lesson on Coping and Defenses!

Meditating on Anger

Many of us have anger toward certain members of our family. Some of us have anger and rage that just seems to go on and on...

For many of us, anger was the only way to break an unhealthy bond or connection between a family member and ourselves. It was the force that kept us from being held captive by certain family members.

It is important for us to allow ourselves to feel and to accept our anger toward family members without casting guilt or shame on ourselves. It is also important to examine our guilty feelings, because anger and guilt are often intertwined.

Let us be as angry as we need to be right now. Thank goodness for the feelings. Feel them. We can accept, even thank, our anger for protecting us. And let us release this anger in healthy ways.

At some point, strive to be done with the anger. As long as we hold on to anger and resentment, it has power over us. We can set a new goal: taking our freedom. Once we do, we won't need our anger anymore. Once we do, we can achieve forgiveness.

We can then replace angry thoughts in a conscious way with loving, healing thoughts toward our family members. We ask our Higher Power to help us grasp freedom and take care of ourselves. Let the golden light of healing shine upon all we love and upon all with whom we feel anger. Let the golden light of healing shine upon us, too.

Trust that a healing is taking place, now.

Help me accept the potent emotions I may feel toward family members. Help me be grateful for the lessons they are teaching me. I accept the golden light of healing that is now shining on my family and me. I accept that healing does not always come in a neat, tidy package.

Note: One good way to be done with anger is to write down what makes us most angry and then talk about it with a safe person. This allows us to <u>acknowledge</u> our anger (writing it down) and to <u>verify and connect</u> it to the real world (talking it over).

Defense and Defensiveness

What is the difference between a defense and defensiveness?

A defense is a method we may use to protect ourselves.

Being defensive is being prepared to defend ourselves, expecting an attack. If we act defensively, always expecting an attack on us, we may miss opportunities for positive interaction with others which is the lifeblood of healthy living.

CHILL

Straight Talk About Stress

C.   Communicate your needs

H.   Health through exercise

I.   Image – strengthen your self-image with positives

L.   Lighten up

L.   Little by Little

My Thoughts Affect Me

1. What negative things do I believe about myself?

2. Are these negatives motivated by other people, by my own fears and moods, or by something I have actually done or that was done to me?

   Deconstruct each negative thing:

   - Is it really true?
   - Why or why not?
   - How can I reverse this negative view of myself?
   - Do I have to change my actions?
   - Do I have to change my thinking?
   - Do I need to make amends to another?
   - What can I do if another will not accept amends from me?
   - Does another owe amends to me?
   - What can I do if another who owes amends does not make them?

3. My thinking affects my feelings, so

   - What are my blessings? What am I grateful for?
   - Let me recount my accomplishments.
   - What are my good traits?
   - What do I like about myself and what do others like about me?

4. Am I lovable?

5. Am I capable of giving love?

6. Am I capable of taking in love?

Families Having a Hard Time Talking

What are some of the reasons families have a hard time talking with one another? Possible answers include:

- There is not enough time together because family members stay away from home a lot.
- Time together is often spent in activities that do not allow for much talking, such as watching TV.
- Sometimes family talks become arguments.
- Some parents may be drinking and children are afraid to talk to them.
- Some parents do not feel children should be listened to; they should be "seen and not heard."
- Sometimes parents come from families where talking about difficult subjects was never done and so they don't know how to do it for themselves or to model it for their children.

Explain to the children that to be an effective communicator with your family and friends you need to abide by some rules such as:

- One person talks at a time.
- Everyone gets a chance to talk.
- Do not talk while another person is talking.
- Do not say that another person's ideas are dumb.
- Use "I" statements.

Have your children complete the "I Feel" Messages that follow, looking for volunteers but choosing so that all children participate if possible. Then you and your children commit to practicing these skills at home all the time.

Convert the messages below from "you" messages to "I feel" messages:

- You make me mad when you take my pencil
- You make me sad when you say those things
- You make me happy when you smile
- You made me do that
- You make me angry when you do that
- You make me sick when you throw food
- It's your fault I have to stay after school
- You made me get into trouble

Answers:

- I feel annoyed when you take my pencil
- I feel sad when you say those things
- I feel happy when I see you smile
- I feel that your action caused me to do that
- I feel angry when you do that
- I feel upset when you throw food
- I feel unfriendly toward you because I have to stay after school
- I feel angry because what you did got me into trouble

Remember, nobody can argue with your statement about how you feel.

A more complete approach to the "I" statement is to do the following:

- I want to talk to you about what you did yesterday.
- (If this is an adult) Is this a good time to talk about it? (if not, agree on a time)
- Do you remember knocking over the vase while you were running in the house?
- I feel frustrated about it because we have often talked about this, and you agreed not to do it
- What do you think we should do so it won't happen again?

Note: a consequence should be proportionate to the severity of the transgression and related to the action where possible. A child will often suggest a consequence that is too severe. Be sure to make an adjustment to the consequence to keep it proportionate, and alter the consequence if necessary to make it more directly connected to the action.

Lesson Four: What is a Drug?

<u>Objectives:</u>   Children ...

1. learn the definition of a drug
2. learn to recognize the effects of some drugs, including tobacco, alcohol and marijuana
3. become aware of the safe uses of drugs
4. become aware that chemical dependency (including alcoholism) is a disease
5. learn that chemical dependency is a disease that is chronic and progressive, and what these words mean
   - chronic = "once you've got it, you've got it for good"
   - progressive="symptoms just keep getting worse as long as use continues"

<u>Key Messages:</u>

A drug is any substance that changes the way our body or our mind works. There are safe and unsafe drugs. There are legal and illegal drugs.

Safe drugs include over the counter drugs such as aspirin and cough medicine and well as prescription drugs, which are supplied by the pharmacist to us based on a doctor's prescription. All safe drugs can be unsafe if not used properly, that is, when not needed, in the wrong amount, if used too long or not long enough, if used at the wrong time of day or the wrong number of times per day, if prescribed for someone else, or if outdated.

Unsafe drugs are all drugs purchased on the street as well as alcohol (for some people) and tobacco. Street drugs such as marijuana, cocaine, heroin, amphetamines, crack, methamphetamines, etc. are addictive. That means that people who use them run a strong risk of not being able to stop using, once they have started. While this is commonly called addiction, people in the medical community call addiction by another term, namely 'chemical dependency'.

Chemically Dependency is a disease because it has a defined set of symptoms and it responds to treatment. People who are chemically dependent are responsible for taking care of themselves and staying healthy, the same as people who have other medical conditions, such as diabetes or heart disease. If a person has addiction in his or her family, especially if a lot of close relatives are chemically dependent, then that person has a much higher risk of becoming addicted if he or she begins using alcohol or other drugs. The same applies if someone begins using drugs in his or her early teens even if no one in the family is chemically dependent. No one who is chemically dependent ever dreamed he or she would become addicted when starting to use alcohol or other drugs.

Some drugs are mind-altering (those which cause physical changes in the brain such as alcohol, marijuana, cocaine, amphetamines, heroin, etc.) while others are mood-altering (such as caffeine and nicotine). People who are chemically dependent cannot use any mind-altering drug without an immediate serious medical effect called 'relapse'.

No one can use nicotine (smoke or chew tobacco) for a long period without serious medical effects. However, nicotine will not cause a chemically dependent person to relapse. Tobacco is an example of a drug that is legal but unsafe and addictive. Alcohol is unsafe if used irresponsibly and for some people it is addictive. Young people cannot use nicotine or alcohol legally until they are 18 and 21 years old, respectively. The drug that causes people the most death and destruction is alcohol because it is the most widely used.

This lesson can be nicely approached by asking a series of questions:

What is a drug? (anything we put into our ourselves that changes the way our bodies or minds work)

Are all drugs harmful? (no, prescription drugs and over the counter are safe when used correctly)

Are all drugs addictive? (no – examples are Tylenol, Motrin, antibiotics, etc.)

What do we call the drugs we buy in drugstores ? (over-the-counter if not prescribed by a doctor, prescription drugs from pharmacy)

Who provides us with prescription drugs? (a licensed pharmacist)

Can over-the-counter drugs harm us? (yes - misuse, wrong dosage, wrong person, "adult only" when taken by child, out of date)

Can prescription drugs harm us? (yes, misuse, wrong dosage, wrong person, out of date)

Are all illegal drugs harmful? (yes)

Name some types of drugs that people use to alter their minds (thinking) and their moods. (Alcohol, marijuana, cocaine, pain pills, heroin, ecstasy, LSD, methamphetamine, inhalants, GHB, PCP, club drugs)

Are all illegal drugs addictive? (yes)

What is the difference between 'Mind Altering' and 'Mood Altering' drugs? (Mind-altering drugs actually change the structure of the brain. They also can cause chemical dependency, or addiction. When taken by a person with addiction who is in recovery, i.e., not using, they will cause a relapse. On the other hand, tobacco (although it is harmful) is a mood altering drug that can be used without causing relapse.)

What is relapse? (a relapse is a resumption of drug use by an addict after a time of non-use)

What is recovery? (recovery is when an addicted person gets medical and psychological help and is able to stop using all mind-altering drugs)

What are some mind altering drugs? (alcohol, marijuana, cocaine, pain pills, heroin, ecstasy, LSD, meth amphetamines, inhalants, GHB, PCP, club drugs,...)

What are some mood altering drugs? (tobacco/nicotine, coffee/caffeine,...)

Are mood altering drugs safe? (tobacco is not safe for anyone)

Can tobacco cause damage to someone who doesn't use it? What is this damage called? (yes, second-hand smoke damage)

What drug causes more illness and death than all the others combined? (alcohol, because it's used by more people)

Is alcohol legal? At what age? (yes, but only for people over 21 years old)

Is alcohol a mind-altering drug? (yes, it becomes one at the time of addiction. Although many people can use it without difficulty, it can't be used by people in recovery without causing relapse.)

Can some people use alcohol without becoming addicted? (yes, most people can. However, everyone's tolerance is different and no one knows how much a given person can use before becoming addicted. Approximately one out of every ten people who drinks becomes addicted to it.)

What can happen to people who use too much alcohol but don't become addicted? (risky behavior, rape, car crashes, legal problems, drunk driving arrests, family problems, work or school problems, violence, unintended pregnancy, embarrassment, ...)

What about those who do become addicted? (all of the

above, plus cirrhosis of the liver, overdose - which is called alcohol poisoning, and the addiction itself, which if untreated often leads to incarceration or to an early death.)

<u>Is alcoholism one kind of chemical dependency</u>? (yes)

<u>Are children who use alcohol at greater risk of developing alcoholism than people who start using alcohol when they are adults</u>? (yes, children who begin drinking before age 15 are four times more likely to develop alcoholism than those who begin at age 21. You should also know the brain doesn't finish development until age 26, so the risk continues to decline the longer one puts off drinking up to this age.)

<u>Are children of families with high rates of addiction more likely to become addicted themselves</u>? (yes, if they start using their risks are much higher; however, there is no way to predict who will become addicted and how much usage will lead a given person to fall into addiction. It is important for children to hear that no one at all ever needs to become addicted if he or she makes a decision to never use mind-altering drugs. There are many people at high genetic risk who have chosen this path.)

<u>How many alcoholics thought they would become addicted when they started experimenting with alcohol</u>? (not one)

Why do you think young people start experimenting with alcohol and other drugs? (curiosity, peer pressure, uncomfortable feelings, advertising, feels good, ...you tell us)

What is a hookah? (it is a water pipe, like a bong, used to smoke tobacco)

Is smoking through a hookah more or less harmful than a cigarette? (more harmful; smoking tobacco through a hookah for 30 minutes is like smoking 100 cigarettes; also, it is suspected that hookah smoking may be the leading cause of new cases of tuberculosis, a dangerous, life-threatening lung disease, because of bacteria in the tubes and hoses attached to the hookah)

How does alcohol affect people? (it changes the way we feel, to relax us and lower inhibitions, it can harm our liver and other organs, it can cause us to act differently or take risks, it slows down reaction time, it reduces coordination, it causes weight gain, it unbalances diet,...)

Are there 'hard drugs' and 'soft drugs'? (no, while many people think drugs like heroin or cocaine are much worse than alcohol or marijuana, a person's brain doesn't know the difference and all mind-altering drugs can cause addiction)

<u>What has more alcohol in it?</u>

- a can of beer
- a shot of whiskey
- a glass of wine

(all three have about the same amount of alcohol and therefore the same effect on a person's blood alcohol content)

Activities

Feelings Bag – as described in Lesson Two (recommended for each lesson)

Purpose: for children to learn that we can ease the burden of uncomfortable feelings just by talking about them.

Circle Ball Toss – (works best for larger groups) with a supply of soft balls or small stuffed animals at hand, stand in a circle and start to gently toss a ball or animal around. The idea is for us as a group to keep the ball going without dropping it to the floor. After a short while a second ball or animal is added, then a third, and so on. Soon there is chaos and many balls and stuffed animals are dropping to the floor. This game shows what it's like when a person is addicted to drugs. As one uses more and more drugs to get the same effect, one fails to meet more and more of life's responsibilities and eventually one's life is in chaos.

Purpose: children learn that as people use more and more illegal (mind altering) drugs, their lives become ever more chaotic.

Myth and Fact – each participant, including parents, writes two or three things that some people believe to be true of drugs on sticky notes. Then, as a group, we decide which things are true (facts) and which are not true (myths). A worksheet is included in the Supplemental materials at the end of this lesson.

Purpose: children learn that many people think things are

true about drugs, that in fact are not true.

Drug Jeopardy – each child (or team) in turn selects jeopardy questions from categories and gains points for correct answers. Jeopardy sheets for the game are included for common drugs in the Supplemental materials at the end of this lesson. Choose categories for the game that would naturally be interesting to children in your group according to their age and experience.

Purpose: children learn many facts about drugs.

Journals – children write how drugs have affected them or someone close to them (among family or friends).

Purpose: children learn that many people are touched by drug abuse and addiction.

Rag Banners – the parent provides light-colored rags for the children to decorate with anti-drug affirmations and slogans, such as Hugs not Drugs, Free to Be Me, etc. Some fabric markers are permanent so be careful in their use.

Purpose: children learn that a drug-free life is fun.

Tangle – (for larger groups) Parents and children form a circle and each person holds with the right hand the right hand of another person who is not standing alongside. Doing the same with the left hand, each person chooses someone different to hold left hands with. Then everyone tries to get untangled without letting go hands.

Purpose: children learn that tangled lives can be sorted out.

Pillowcases – parents provide an inexpensive white pillowcase for each participant (which includes the parents). Participants use fabric markers to decorate their pillowcases with anti-drug slogans (for example: "Don't Choose Booze", "Smoke's No Joke", and so on). Encourage the children create their own slogans. At the end, participants take turns showing off their artwork and ability to create interesting slogans. Praise is given generously.

Purpose: Our pillowcases protect our pillows, keeping them safe and clean from outside things and they are a comfortable place to rest our heads. Symbolically, they represent us protecting ourselves by making healthy choices that reduce the likelihood of negative consequences. (Note - rather than just stating all this, it is better if the parent starts off by asking the children why they did this exercise, what the pillowcases might represent symbolically. You will likely get many interesting and insightful ideas.)

Journaling

The single recommended topic for today's lesson is:

- "How have drugs affected you or someone you know ?"

When everyone is finished (including the parents), we may share what we have written.

Review – What is a Drug?

1. What is a drug? (answer – anything that changes the way our body or our mind works)
2. Are there safe and unsafe drugs (answer – yes)
3. What are some safe drugs? (answer – aspirin, cough medicine, antibiotics, ...)
4. When are safe drugs not safe? (answer – if we take it when we don't need it, if we take too much or too little, if we take someone else's drug, if we don't take a drug as long as we are supposed to)
5. Where can we buy safe drugs? (answer – at a drug store/pharmacy)
6. What kind of paper do you need to get a drug from the pharmacist? (answer – a prescription)
7. What are these drugs called? (answer – prescription drugs)
8. Who writes the prescription? (answer – a doctor)
9. Who fills the prescription? (answer – a pharmacist)
10. What are the drugs called that you buy from a drug store shelf? (answer – Over-the-Counter drugs)
11. Why are some drugs called "street drugs"? (answer – they are sold illegally on the streets)
12. What are some street drugs? (answer – marijuana, cocaine, Vicodin, heroin,...)
13. Which street drugs can you get in a pharmacy? (answer – none)
14. Are any street drugs safe to use? Which ones? (answer – none)
15. Why not? (answer – you don't know what is in them,

you could overdose and die, you could be arrested, you could cause a car crash, you could become addicted,...)

16. Which legal drugs are risky to use? (answer – alcohol and tobacco)

17. Why are they risky? (answer – liver disease, heart disease, lung/throat/mouth cancer, alcohol overdose which is called alcohol poisoning, risky behavior with alcohol, addiction,...)

18. What can a person who is drunk do to sober up more quickly? (answer – absolutely nothing, only the passage of time sobers a person up)

19. What are the legal ages to buy alcohol and tobacco? (answer – 21 and 18 years old)

20. How old will you be when your brain first reaches full development? (answer – age 26)

21. Is it riskier to use alcohol or other drugs before your brain is fully developed? (answer – yes)

22. Why is it very risky to use alcohol or other drugs at an early age? (answer – the chances of becoming addicted are much higher, our brain's capability to exercise good judgment is not fully formed leading to risky behavior, ...)

23. What does 'Chemical Dependency' mean? (answer – addiction to alcohol or other drugs)

24. What is a person called who is chemically dependent on alcohol? (answer – an alcoholic)

25. Can people who are chemically dependent stop using on their own? (answer – most can't)

26. Are chemically dependent people who keep on using just lazy? (answer – no, they include people who have worked hard all their lives, for example, doctors,

lawyers, judges, police officers, school teachers, people from every walk of life)

27. What program do chemically dependent people follow to stop using alcohol and other drugs? (answer – many use a 12-step program)

28. Are there 'hard' and 'soft' drugs? And if there are, which are hard and which are soft? (answer – there are no hard and soft drugs. They all affect the brain. Our brain doesn't know the difference.)

29. Why do young people experiment with drugs? (answer – peer pressure, curiosity, boredom, desire to get high, wanting to bury uncomfortable feelings,...)

30. Is chemically dependency a disease? (answer – yes, it has symptoms and it responds to treatment)

31. Do chemically dependent parents, who continue to use, love their children? (answer – yes, but the drug is in control so they often can't show their love)

Homework

Name a safe drug (when used as directed)

Name a drug that is legal but always unsafe

Name a drug that is illegal but safe (trick question!)

Name a drug that is legal but unsafe for some people

What mind-altering drug causes more deaths than any other drug?

Homework Answers

Name a safe drug (when used as directed) – aspirin

Name a drug that is legal but always unsafe – nicotine

Name a drug that is illegal but safe (trick question!) – none

Name a drug that is legal but unsafe for some people – alcohol

What mind-altering drug causes more deaths than any other drug – alcohol, because more people use it

The Seven C's

The Seven C's goes like this:

You didn't **C**ause it

You can't **C**ure it

You can't **C**ontrol it

But you **C**an take care of yourself, by

Making healthy **C**hoices for yourself

Communicating your feelings, and

Celebrating who you are

What I Liked Best About Today

Ask your child,

What did you like best about today?

Did you enjoy the time we spent together?

What is one important thing you learned today that you

didn't know before?

Serenity Pledge

Grant me the Serenity to accept the

people I cannot change,

The Courage to change the person I can,

And the Wisdom to know that person is me!

- This ends today's lesson on What is a
Drug?

Myth or Fact

Above are some common mistaken ideas about alcoholism.
Draw a line from each Myth to its corresponding Fact.

Myths

Alcoholism is only a bad habit.

A child can make his mother not drink if he makes his bed every day.

A person who goes to work is not an alcoholic.

Not many children have an alcoholic parent.

Children can cause their parents to drink too much by being bad.

A person who drinks only wine or beer is not an alcoholic.

Children of alcoholics should only get help if their parent stops drinking.

Women can't become alcoholics.

Alcoholics can never get well.

Facts

Many alcoholics have a job.

Children of alcoholics deserve help for themselves.

Drinking any alcoholic beverage can lead to alcoholism.

Women as well as men can become alcoholics.

Children cannot cause their parents to drink too much.

Children cannot make their parents stop drinking.

There are seven million children with an alcoholic parent.

Alcoholism is a sickness.

Alcoholics can stop drinking with the proper help.

Are there any myths that you believed were true?
Draw a circle around each one.

Drug Jeopardy – Drugs

- For 100 points: Are all drugs harmful?

answer: no

- For 200 points: Can every drug be harmful if used improperly?

answer: yes

- For 300 points: Name four reasons why teenagers experiment with unsafe drugs.

answer: choose from: peer pressure, desire to fit in, boredom, uncomfortable feelings, low self-esteem, wanting to experience the 'high', advertising (for alcohol and cigarettes), wanting to celebrate

- for 400 points: What organ of the body do all illegal drugs quickly effect?

answer: the brain

- For 500 points: What is a drug?

answer: anything we put into our body that changes the way we feel or think, or the way our body works

- Daily Double: Do different people using the same drug the same way have the same chance of becoming addicted?

answer: no, everyone's brain reacts differently

depending on genetic make-up.

Drug Jeopardy – Legal Drugs

- For 100 points: Are all drugs that are legal for adults to buy also safe for them to use?

answer: no

- For 200 points: Name two drugs that are legal for adults, but not safe to use?

answer: tobacco and (for some people) alcohol

- For 300 points: Where do we buy safe, legal drugs.

answer: drug store/pharmacy

- for 400 points: What are the two categories of drugs found in a drug store?

answer: prescription and over-the-counter

- For 500 points: What are the two main reasons teens misuse prescription drugs?

answer: they are often easily available in the home, and the misconception that because they are medicine, they are safe

- Daily Double: Name a prescription drug that is very addictive?

answer: pain pills

Drug Jeopardy – <u>Illegal Drugs</u>

- For 100 points: How can you be sure what's in a street drug you buy?

answer: you can't – you have absolutely no idea

- For 200 points: What item comes with every item you buy in a store but never with a street drug?

answer: choose from: a guarantee, a receipt

- For 300 points: What is a 'gateway' drug

answer: a drug commonly used early in the use-abuse-addiction cycle

- for 400 points: What are two gateway drugs?

answer: alcohol and marijuana

- For 500 points: What's the difference between a 'hard drug' and a 'soft drug'?

answer: nothing, so-called 'soft' drugs can lead to the same problems as 'hard' drugs, including addiction

- Daily Double: What kind of friends does a person have, who abuses 'street' drugs?

answer: drug-using friends

Drug Jeopardy – <u>Alcohol</u>

- For 100 points: What is the name of the disease when someone can't stop drinking?

answer: alcoholism

- For 200 points: What can you do to sober up someone who has been drinking?

answer: nothing – only the passage of time makes a person sober

- For 300 points: What is 'binge drinking'?

answer: drinking 5 or more drinks in one sitting

- for 400 points: what should you do if you find someone passed out?

answer: call 911

- For 500 points: what are two dangers to a baby if the mother drinks alcohol during pregnancy?

answer: (1) birth defects and (2) fetal alcohol syndrome

- Daily Double: Why is someone who begins using alcohol before age 26 more likely to become an alcoholic?

answer: the person's brain is not fully developed until age 26

Drug Jeopardy – <u>Tobacco</u>

- For 100 points: What is the addictive drug in tobacco?

answer: nicotine

- For 200 points: Name two ways tobacco can be used.

answer: smoked or chewed

- For 300 points: What do we call it when people breathe in other people's exhaled smoke?

answer: second-hand smoke

- for 400 points: Name two diseases caused by tobacco?

answer: choose from: cancer, heart disease, emphysema

- For 500 points: Name two risks for a baby of a mother who smokes during pregnancy?

answer: choose from: lower birth rate, increased risk of infant death, increased risk of childhood cancer

- Daily Double: True or False: tobacco use killed about 100 million people in the 20th century?

answer: true

Drug Jeopardy – <u>Marijuana</u>

- For 100 points: Is marijuana addictive both physically and psychologically?

answer: yes

- For 200 points: Name two effects on a person's body or mind, who regularly smokes marijuana.

answer: choose from: short-term memory loss, cancer, addiction

- For 300 points: One marijuana joint has as many cancer-causing agents as how many cigarettes?

answer: between 3 and 4

- for 400 points: How many chemicals are in a marijuana joint?

answer: over 400

- For 500 points: What are 5 negative non-medical consequences that may occur to someone who uses marijuana?

answer: choose from: family problems, school problems, problems at work, legal problems, car crash, loss of outside interests, impaired decision-making (possibly leading to pregnancy or sexually-transmitted diseases), impaired coordination, loss of motivation and goals

- Daily Double: True or False: marijuana can cause psychosis in those at risk?   (Psychosis is a loss of contact with reality and deterioration in social functioning)

answer: true, in some people marijuana can have this effect

Drug Jeopardy – <u>Prescription Drugs</u>

- For 100 points: What is the difference between a prescription drug and an over-the-counter drug?

answer: you need a doctor's authorization (prescription) to get a prescription drug

- For 200 points: Name two ways an over-the-counter drug may not be safe.

answer: choose from: using too much, using without a need, or using out-of-date drugs

- For 300 points: Name three ways a prescription drug may not be safe?

answer: choose from: using someone else's prescription, using the wrong amount, using for too long or not long enough, using an out-of-date drug

- for 400 points: Why is it not safe to stop using a prescription drug before the prescription runs out?

answer: an infection might not be completely eliminated, and the remaining germs would be likely the most resistant of the bunch, making it harder to kill a resurgence of the infection

For 500 points: What is the name of the first highly effective antibiotic?

answer: penicillin

- Daily Double: Why do researchers continue to develop new types of antibiotics?

answer: because germs develop resistance to antibiotics so older drugs become less effective over time

Drug Jeopardy – <u>Inhalants and Club Drugs</u>

- For 100 points: What are inhalants?

answer: substances found in many household products that can be inhaled to produce a 'high'

- For 200 points: Can a person die from a single prolonged sniffing of an inhalant?

answer: yes

- For 300 points: Which of the following is true? (a) inhalants are extremely toxic, or (b) inhalants can cause brain damage, or (c) inhalants can damage heart, kidneys and lungs, or (d) all of the above

answer: (d),   all of the above

- for 400 points: What club drug may contain heroin, speed and rat poison?

answer: Ecstasy

- For 500 points: Name two ways a 'date-rape' drug might affect your mind?

answer: choose from: confusion, loss of consciousness, distorted memory

- Daily Double: What is the most common 'date-rape' drug?

answer: alcohol

Drug Jeopardy – <u>Amphetamines</u>

- For 100 points: True or false, methamphetamine is one of the amphetamines?

answer: true

- For 200 points: Are amphetamines stimulants or depressants?

answer: stimulants

- For 300 points: True or false, methamphetamines are made of common, toxic household products?

answer: true

- for 400 points: True or false, methamphetamines often result in disfigurement?

answer: true

- For 500 points: What are two feelings amphetamines produce?

answer: euphoria and alertness

- Daily Double: True or false, methamphetamine is extremely addictive and has permanent health effects?

answer: true

Drug Jeopardy – <u>Heroin</u>

- For 100 points: True or false, one can become addicted to heroin the first time using?

answer: true

- For 200 points: True or false, one can die the first time using heroin?

answer: true

- For 300 points: True or false, heroin is a 'hard' drug?

answer: false, there is no distinction between the so-called 'hard' and 'soft' drugs as they are all mind-altering and can lead to addiction.   However, heroin is extremely dangerous and is one of the top two frequently reported drugs cited by medical examiners in drug abuse deaths.

- for 400 points: What are two ways heroin may be used?

answer: choose from: injecting, snorting, smoking

- For 500 points: True or false, withdrawal from heroin can kill you?

answer: false.   Withdrawal is seldom fatal but is exceedingly uncomfortable. It is highly recommended to go through withdrawal in a medical facility.

- Daily Double: True or false, heroin is less dangerous if you snort or smoke it instead of injecting it?

answer: false.   Heroin is heroin. There is no safe way to ingest it. You can still die from an overdose or become addicted by snorting or smoking it.

Drug Jeopardy – <u>Cocaine</u>

- For 100 points: True or false, even a first-time user can die of a heart attack or seizure?

answer: true

- For 200 points: Name two ways a person's body or mind is affected by cocaine.

answer: choose from: increased heart rate, damaged nasal tissues, muscle spasms, convulsions, irregular eating and sleeping, short-lived 'high', addiction

- For 300 points: What are three ways cocaine can be used?

answer: snorted, injected, smoked

- for 400 points: What are two ways cocaine can kill you?

answer: choose from: heart attack, stroke, seizure, respiratory failure, as well as (from sharing needles) HIV/AIDS and Hepatitis C

- For 500 points: After the cocaine 'high' passes, how does a person often feel? Name five ways.

answer: choose from: depressed, uninterested, isolated, shamed, guilty, out of control, edgy, anxious, angry, hostile, craving (for more of the drug)

- Daily Double: True or false, people convicted of using

'crack' are currently sentenced to longer jail time than users of powdered cocaine?

answer: true, although efforts are underway to equalize sentencing

Drug Jeopardy – Hallucinogens

- For 100 points: True or false, hallucinogens can make a person see things and hear voices that don't exist?

answer: true

- For 200 points: Name two ways hallucinogens affect a person's heart.

answer: increased heart rate and increased blood pressure

- For 300 points: True or false, hallucinogens can cause flashback and hallucinations months or years after one's last use?

answer: true

- for 400 points: Which of these things can hallucinogens cause a person to do? (a) mix up speech, (b) lose muscle control, (c) act aggressively, irrationally and violently, or (d) all of these things?

answer: (d), all of these things

- For 500 points: What are three warning signs a friend may be using hallucinogens?

answer: choose from: distorted senses (time, space, sight, hearing, touch), dilated pupils, anxiety, paranoia, irrational behavior, mood swings, fainting

- Daily Double: What percentage of teens have ever tried hallucinogens? (a) 1%   (b) 6% or   (c) 18%

answer: (b), 6 % according to a 2002 study

Where Do I Stand?

Mark somewhere on the line where you stand on each statement

I would drink alcohol rather than be called a chicken.   Y_____Maybe_____N

I would take a friend's prescription pain pill if my tooth hurt a lot.   Y_____Maybe_____N

I think marijuana should be legalized.
Y_____Maybe_____N

I think all public buildings should be smoke free.
Y_____Maybe_____N

I think people who smoke in nonsmoking areas should be fined.   Y_____Maybe_____N

I think the legal drinking age should be 21.
Y_____Maybe_____N

I'd report someone who is selling marijuana at my school.
Y_____Maybe_____N

I'd report someone who is selling cocaine at my school.

Y_____Maybe_____N

I think drinking at weekend parties is okay.
Y_____Maybe_____N

I'd tell my parents if my sister or brother was abusing
alcohol or other drugs.   Y_____Maybe_____N

I think you can have more fun without alcohol or other
drugs.   Y_____Maybe_____N

Lesson Five: Stages of Dependency

<u>Goals</u>:   Children ...

1.   are reminded that alcoholism and other drug addiction is a progressive disease with different stages of dependency that increase in severity
2.   are reminded that alcoholism and other drug addiction is a chronic disease, which means it can be managed (through recovery) but not cured
3.   realize that someone else's addiction is not their fault
4.   learn that it's okay for them to ask for help even if the chemically dependent family member does not get help
5.   realize there are safe places and people to turn to for help
6.   realize that if they live in a family with addiction, they are not alone
7.   learn that if they live in a family with addiction, they may be at higher risk of addiction than their peers, because addiction tends to run in families

<u>Key Messages</u>:

Alcoholism and other drug addiction is a disease. It is chronic and progressive. *Chronic* means that once a person becomes chemically dependent she/he will always be chemically dependent. It can't be cured. *Progressive* means that if a person with the disease keeps using, his/her physical and mental condition will get worse and worse.

If someone in our family is addicted it is never our fault. Sometime the addicted person may say it's our fault, but it's not. We didn't cause that person to start using, we don't cause him or her to continue to use, and we can't do anything to make things better for that person no matter how much we do or how hard we try. We can't cure the disease nor can we control its effects on the person we love. However, we can learn to take care of ourselves by making healthy choices for ourselves, communicating our feelings and celebrating who we are.

One healthy choice we can make is to *not enable*. Enabling is when we try to fix the problems that another person is causing for him- or herself that come from using alcohol or other drugs. Enabling never works - in fact it makes the problem worse.

It's not selfish for us to enjoy our lives even though a loved one may be suffering with addiction. In fact, by taking care of ourselves and enjoying our lives we are at least setting a good example for others in our family. Often family members need help to deal with all the pain that has been caused by the addiction of their loved one. There are programs for family members such as 12-step Al Anon and Alateen, school programs, and hospital-run summer camps that help with these issues.

There are three *stages* of chemical dependency. These are stages that all chemically dependent people have passed through. The first is the *learning stage*, where a person experiments with alcohol or other drugs because of peer pressure, curiosity, or for some other reason. A person in the learning stage is not (yet) chemically dependent and can't imagine that he or she ever will be. If use continues long enough, the person will enter the *seeking stage*, where one's life is organized around using opportunities. For example, one may choose only restaurants that serve alcohol as places to go for dining. The third stage is the *loss of choice* stage. In this stage one is no longer able to stop using by oneself. The person needs help and help is found in *recovery*.

Activities

Feelings Bag – as described in Lesson Two (recommended for each lesson)

Purpose: for children to learn that we can ease the burden of uncomfortable feelings just by talking about them.

Rad Ads – Parents and children together go through a stack of old magazines, cutting out advertisements for tobacco, wine, vodka, prescription and non-prescription medications, and other drug-related ads and pasting or taping them to sheets of paper. Parents and children discuss how the advertisements are intended to motivate people to buy and use these products. The visual messages of glamour and fun associated with cigarettes and alcohol products are discussed with special emphasis to show how advertising is used to get people to use these drugs more than they might otherwise do. Children are asked if people would buy these products as readily if they didn't have the fun/glamour signals attached. Children are asked if people who use these products more than most are likely to look like the people in the ads. Ask the children, "What do the words in the advertisement say?" Then ask them, "What does the picture say?" Ask them whether the words and the picture are saying the same things. Ask how children can protect themselves against the picture's message. (*answer:* awareness)

Purpose: to demonstrate to the child that many millions of dollars are spent each year to influence people to use drug products, and that these advertising dollars are more than paid off by profits from the additional sales of the product.

Journals - write about a time you made a decision to not use tobacco, alcohol or other drugs OR about a problem in your family that's related to alcohol or other drug use OR about a problem in another family that you know. At the end, we have a chance to share what we have written.

Purpose: to understand how alcohol or other drugs have affected us and other people we know.

Stages of Dependency Jeopardy – each child (or team) selects jeopardy questions from categories and gains points for correct answers. Jeopardy sheets for the game are included for the stages of sependency in the Supplemental materials at the end of this lesson.

Purpose: children learn how chemical dependency develops through stages of dependency.

Snowball Fight – (for larger groups) all participants write three things about themselves that most people don't know, on a piece of paper. Then all crumple up their sheets and have a one minute snowball fight. (Make sure everyone understands not to throw at anyone else's face.) At the end of one minute each person picks up a 'snowball' and goes around trying to find out whose snowball it is. Then each participant introduces the snowball person to the rest of the group.

Purpose: to get to know something new about one another.

Line in the Sand – put a long piece of masking tape along the floor, creating a tightrope. You have to work hard to keep your balance. Then parents gently toss soft toys at the child, making it even more difficult. Parents ask the children what these soft toys represent (life's difficulties). Ask the child to bend down and pick up a soft toy lying near the tape. Ask if this is difficult and what picking up the toy represents (extra effort that someone in early recovery must make to stay on the path to recovery).

Purpose: to understand life's challenges are to be met with calm determination.

Journaling

Some suggested topics for this lesson are:

1. "One time I made a decision to not use tobacco, alcohol or other drugs was ..."

2. "The biggest problem in our family, that's related to someone's use of alcohol or other drugs, is ..."

3. "There's a big problem in a family, not my own, that I know about. The problem is..."

Often, we give the child a choice of topics. When everyone is finished (including the parent), we may share what we have written.

Review – Stages of Dependency

1. Is chemical dependency a disease? (answer – yes, it has symptoms and it can be treated)
2. What is the difference between addiction and chemical dependency (answer – no difference, they are the same thing)
3. Can anyone become chemically dependent? (answer – yes, if a person uses)
4. What are the risk factors for becoming addicted? (answer – how early one starts using, how much the person uses, and family history)
5. Is alcohol a drug? (answer – yes, it is a mind-altering drug)
6. Name some mind-altering drugs (answer – alcohol, marijuana, pain pills, glue, amphetamines, meth, crystal meth, cocaine, crack, heroin, PCP, peyote, ecstasy and many more)
7. Name some mood-altering drugs (answer – the most common are nicotine and caffeine)
8. What plant is nicotine found in? (answer – tobacco leaf)
9. What plant is caffeine found in? (answer – coffee bean)
10. Can people become addicted to mood-altering drugs? (answer – yes, millions are addicted to nicotine)
11. Why is a mind-altering drug different from a mood-altering drug (answer – a mind-altering drug makes permanent physical and chemical changes in the brain. Also, an addict cannot use a mind-altering drug without relapsing.)
12. What are the three stages of chemical dependency?

(answer – the learning stage, the seeking stage and the loss-of-choice stage)

13. What does the learning stage look like? (answer – people use to get high with their friends)

14. If someone in the learning or seeking stage is caught using, can he or she go to jail? (answer – yes)

15. Can he or she suddenly need long-term hospitalization? (answer – yes)

16. Can he or she overdose and die? (answer – with most mind-altering chemicals, yes. Also, the person could crash a car or engage in other risky behavior, e.g., jumping off a hotel balcony toward a swimming pool, which could lead to death)

17. What does the loss-of-choice stage look like? (answer – people use to feel normal and can't stop without help)

18. If someone becomes chemically dependent, is the situation hopeless? (answer - no)

19. What can that person do? (answer – get into treatment and recovery)

20. Doctors use two words to describe the disease of chemical dependency. What are they? (answer – chronic and progressive)

21. What does chronic mean? (answer – once you've got it, you've got it – there's no cure, only disease management, i.e., recovery)

22. What does progressive mean? (answer – with continued use, the condition just keeps getting worse, our physical and mental states continue to deteriorate)

23. What specifically can family members do to help a

chemically dependent loved one?   (answer – follow the Seven C's, namely assuring ourselves as often as necessary that we didn't cause it and we can't control it or cure it, but we can take care of ourselves by making healthy choices, communicating our feelings and celebrating who we are. One of the most helpful choices we can make is to stop enabling, that is, taking away negative consequences, for a loved one who is using.)

24. What does enabling look like? (answer – giving money to the using one, lying for him or her, bailing out of jail, paying for lawyers, or otherwise supporting the unhealthy lifestyle)

25. Is it all right to be angry with a family member who is chemically dependent? (answer – of course, your feelings are your own. We can own our anger and hold our loved one responsible for his/her using actions, while at the same time, if we choose to, we can hold ourselves open to feelings of compassion and understanding. However, if we express our feelings to the chemically dependent family member, as to anyone else, we must do so appropriately.)

26. What does 'letting go' mean? Does it mean we give up on our loved one? (answer – no, it means we set aside our pain, fear, frustration, hurt, anger and other uncomfortable feelings and hand them over to a higher power for safekeeping, so that we can begin to heal ourselves. This is our recovery.)

27. If a friend or family member is chemically dependent and continues to use, what can we do? (answer – we can stop enabling, we can arrange a professional intervention, we can take care of ourselves, and if we choose to and financing is adequate, we can offer to pay for treatment)

28. What is enabling? (answer – it is taking away the consequences of using from the person who is using)

29. What is professional intervention? (answer – it is an event run by a trained professional that involves both the addict and his family and friends. The family and friends tell the addict in a loving but very honest and firm way what they see going on and how it has hurt them. They urge the addict to go into treatment immediately. If the addict agrees, he or she is taken immediately to a treatment center.)

30. Why is taking care of ourselves important? (answer – addiction is called a 'family disease' because all family members are affected. Children may have been ignored or abused. Everyone may be depressed or despondent. Everyone needs and deserves to get help)

31. When family members do get help, what are seven important things they learn? (answer – they learn that they didn't cause the disease their loved one has, they can't control the disease and they can't cure their loved one. But they can start to take care of themselves by making healthy choices, communicating their feelings with safe people and celebrating who they are)

Homework

Pay attention to what you are feeling without any judgment; notice it (hand on heart) and feel it

The Seven C's

The Seven C's goes like this:

You didn't **C**ause it

You can't **C**ure it

You can't **C**ontrol it

But you **C**an take care of yourself, by

Making healthy **C**hoices for yourself

Communicating your feelings, and

Celebrating who you are

What I Liked Best About Today

Ask your child,

What did you like best about today?

Did you enjoy the time we spent together?

What is one important thing you learned today that you

didn't know before?

Serenity Pledge

Grant me the Serenity to accept the

people I cannot change,

The Courage to change the person I can,

And the Wisdom to know that person is me!

- This ends today's lesson on Stages of
Dependency

Stages of Dependency

Every child is curious, occasionally bored, and sometimes troubled by uncomfortable feelings. Children are also social and want to fit in with their friends. A child may choose to experiment with alcohol or other drugs for any of these (or other) reasons, and if so these are the Stages of Dependency the child faces ...

The Learning Stage

For simplicity's sake, let's assume we are talking about a teenage girl.

The Learning stage _feels_ like this: this teenage girl believes that using alcohol or other drugs is fun and that they make her feel better. She finds that using numbs some uncomfortable feelings she has. Sometimes using helps her to temporarily forget her problems.

The Learning stage _looks_ like this: she finds acceptance with using friends but loses some of her old friends. She may face family, school and legal problems and may find herself engaging in risky behaviors.

Some teens may move from the learning stage to ...

The Seeking Stage

The Seeking stage _feels_ like this: our teenage girl now looks forward to using drugs, having learned that drugs affect how she feels.

The Seeking stage _looks_ like this: she now arranges her life around using opportunities. She loses longtime friends and spends time with other users. She starts to become socially isolated and loses what used to be her keenest interests. She has problems with her family and with school and work. She may face legal problems.

Many in the seeking stage move to ...

The Loss of Choice (Addiction) Stage

The Loss of Choice stage _feels_ like this: A chemical change occurs in the girl's body. She can no longer choose whether or not to use, or how much to use. Also, she loses the ability to handle her feelings.

The Loss of Choice stage _looks_ like this: our teen is failing in school and unable to hold a job. She spends all her time either using her drug of choice or focused on getting a new supply. Her feelings are mostly shame, guilt and depression. She is in legal trouble and has extreme family problems. If she is married, her marriage is breaking down and she is losing emotional contact with her children. She has lost the trust of parents, brothers and sisters. She has ever more serious health and emotional problems.

Signs of a Developing Problem with Alcohol

(General Sequence with Minor Variations by Individual)

- drinks with friends
- knows when to stop
- is able to stop
- sometimes is affected by peer pressure

- drinks with strangers (bars, etc.)
- increased tolerance (more alcohol needed for the same "high")
- sometimes continues drinking beyond "planned high"
- risky behaviors, consequences occasionally exceed benefits

- first period of alcohol induced amnesia ("blackout", that is, drinking and related activities continue for a period of which the person has no recollection afterward)
- beginning to "sneak" drinks, awareness that others might notice a problem
- activities begin to be organized around drinking opportunities
- denial takes the form of comparing drinking habits to those of others worse off

----

- drinking becomes a preoccupation, on the mind most of the time
- binge drinking begins (large quantities in one sitting, gulping drinks)
- loss of control (can no longer accurately predict when drinking will stop)

- loss of old friends, new drinking friends
- often drinks alone
- isolates by choice and lifestyle
- consequences routinely exceed benefits

- denial takes the form of stopping for short periods to convince self everything is under control
- may switch from alcohol to another drug
- deterioration of self-esteem and appearance
- deep-seated depression
- personality changes
- health problems, job problems, family problems, legal problems

----

- admits defeat, accepts alcohol's central place in life, refuses to give it up
- makes sure alcohol is always within easy reaching distance

- drinks to relieve withdrawal symptoms
- meaningful life ends

Stages of Dependency Jeopardy –
Addiction/Recovery I

- For 100 points: What is another common term for Chemical Dependency?

answer: addiction

- For 200 points: When a child starts to experiment with alcohol or other drugs, what are some of the consequences he/she will likely face from family, school, and the legal system? Name one from each.

answer: *family* – choose from: loss of trust, restriction; *school* -   choose from :   suspension, expulsion; *legal* – choose from: arrest, court costs, restrictions

- For 300 points: If someone is addicted and continues to use, what are three likely outcomes?

answer: choose from: jail, long-term hospitalization, insanity, premature death

- for 400 points: Chemical dependency is *chronic* and *progressive*.   What does that mean?

answer: Chronic means it never goes away or gets cured; progressive means it keeps getting worse as long as a person continues to use

- For 500 points: What percentage of people who are chemically dependent can achieve recovery and sobriety?

answer: everyone who is wants recovery can achieve it. Once a person surrenders his/her drug of choice as life partner, the road to recovery is clear, well-traveled and full of support. However, some people do not ever choose to commit to a life without their drug of choice.

- Daily Double: If someone becomes addicted, is the situation hopeless?

answer: no, while there are three stages of chemical dependency that everyone who has become addicted has passed through, the fourth stage (recovery) is always open though not always taken.

Stages of Dependency Jeopardy – Addiction/Recovery II

- For 100 points: Name two genetic (inherited) factors that increase the risk of addiction?

answer: choose from: number of family members who are chemically dependent, whether they are close relatives, the individual's brain structure (ADD, ADHD, depression, mental illness)

- For 200 points: What two environmental risk factors increase the risk of addiction?

answer: choose from: (a) family drug use and other stress, (b) influence of peers (friends and acquaintances), and (c) mother's use of drugs during pregnancy

- For 300 points: What are the three stages of chemical dependency?

answer: the learning stage, the seeking stage, and the loss-of-choice/control (addiction) stage

- for 400 points: What does being in the seeking stage mean?

answer: a person organizes his/her life around using opportunities

- For 500 points: What is the difference between *treatment* and *recovery*?

answer: *treatment* addresses the medical needs surrounding withdrawal, as well as psychological, behavioral and educational needs (also called Cognitive Therapy). It is *short-term*. *Recovery* is living a different kind of life usually centered around the 12 step principles. It is *life-long*.

- Daily Double: What can we do if someone we love is addicted and using?

answer: in general, take care of ourselves by making healthy choices, communicating our feelings and celebrating who we are. Specifically, we can stop enabling, support our loved one's efforts to recover, arrange for a professional 'intervention' (if the family member won't admit the problem and go on his own for treatment), address our own recovery needs as family members affected by addiction, and finally, should we choose to and should finances permit, offer to pay for a treatment opportunity.

Stages of Dependency Jeopardy – Addiction/Recovery III

- For 100 points: If a person relapses, does that mean the end of the person's recovery?

answer: no, as long as the person gets right back to the program with renewed purpose

- For 200 points: What are two powerful myths or misconceptions surrounding chemical dependency that many people believe today?

answer: that chemically dependent people are lacking in willpower and morally flawed

- For 300 points: What are two differences between mind-altering and mood-altering drugs?

answer: (a) a mind-altering drug changes the physical structure of the brain permanently while a mood-altering drug affects mood temporarily, (b) someone who is chemically dependent can use mood-altering drugs (such as caffeine and nicotine) without relapsing, but will relapse if he/she uses any mind-altering drug, even if the drug is different from the person's regular drug of choice

- for 400 points: Define addiction?

answer: a chronic, relapsing brain disease characterized by compulsive drug seeking and use, despite harmful consequences far out of proportion to any benefit gained (the 'high')

- For 500 points: Do you believe chemical dependency is a disease? Why or why not?

answer: It is a disease, because just like any other disease such as heart disease or diabetes, it disrupts the normal, healthy functioning of the underlying organ (brain), it has serious harmful consequences, it is treatable, and if left untreated can last a lifetime. More formally, it is a pathological condition resulting from infection (use), genetic defect (family predisposition), or environmental stress (family or other stress) and it is characterized by an identifiable set of signs or symptoms.

- Daily Double: What are the Seven C's?

answer: I didn't cause it, I can't control it, I can't cure it - but I can take care of myself by making healthy choices, communicating my feelings and celebrating who I am.

Lesson Six: Treatment and Recovery

<u>Goals</u>:   Children learn ...

1.   that treatment helps the addicted person to begin recovery
2.   that even in recovery, the possibility of relapse is always present and that people who relapse are not bad people
3.   that there is only one job for someone who is relapsing – get right back into recovery
4.   that recovery is for both the addict and as well for other family members (different programs)
5.   that recovery is not a selfish program but a program centered around self; that it's not selfish to take care of ourselves – it's the responsible thing to do and sets a good example for everyone around
6.   that it's okay for them to ask for help even if their chemically dependent family member does not get help
7.   there are safe people and places to turn to for help

<u>Key Messages</u>:

Treatment helps the addicted person to begin recovery. The first step is for the person to go to a hospital for *detox*. This is a short treatment (3 to 4 days) that gets the person through the physical withdrawal symptoms. Then the patient enters (based on a professional evaluation and sometimes, unfortunately, insurance coverage) either into an *in-patient* rehab (the person spends days and nights at the facility), an *out-patient* rehab (the patient comes to the facility for a few hours every day or a few times a week, or begins a *12-step* program such as Alcoholics Anonymous (AA). In all these programs, the patient learns what to do to recover from the disease of addiction. He/she learns new skills, is introduced to tools and resources he/she can use to find and maintain *sobriety*, which is the complete avoidance of alcohol or other drugs.

A person who is in recovery and who is tempted to use again has *relapsed*. Relapse usually happens by returning to old thinking patterns or behaviors, before actual drug use begins. It may start with spending time with old using acquaintances or sliding back into thinking about using. There is almost always some relapse behavior or thinking before the person first uses again. Chemically dependent people are taught to recognize these backsliding thoughts and patterns early, before they actually use, and to take action immediately, such as contacting their sponsor and going to more meetings. A *sponsor* is another recovering person who has been in recovery for some time and wants to "give back" by helping others who are newer in recovery.

Full-blown relapse is when a person loses all control and returns to his/her old drug using patterns. When a person in recovery start using again, one returns to the same point in the progression of the disease as one was before entering recovery. Full-blown relapse usually requires another detox in a hospital. Relapse does not make a person a bad person, but the person who has relapsed is responsible for the relapse and anything done while relapsing.

When chemically dependent people do get treatment and are in recovery that does not solve all the family's problems. There may be left over problems (such as legal and financial) from the using days and a lot of pain for family members to deal with. Family rules may change and family members may struggle to understand the new rules and guidelines for survival and growth. When addictive behavior stops, the family may not find healthy ways to function because they may never have experienced a healthy environment with predictable rules and behaviors. Also, the recovering person may need to spend a lot of time in recovery groups, time that the family members, especially children, want more of themselves.

There may still be a great deal of tension in the home and often depression and anger to be addressed. It takes time for family members to forgive and trust the family member in recovery. Helping family members learn to handle these feelings and to take care of themselves is critical. In educational support groups and 12-step programs such as Alateen and Al Anon, family members learn to affirm their own perceptions of reality, trust their own feelings, and discover healthy ways of functioning.

Activities

Feelings Bag – as described in Lesson Two (recommended for each lesson)

Purpose: for children to learn that we can ease the burden of uncomfortable feelings just by talking about them.

Tangle Knots – we make a messy group and hold hands randomly, each person holding hands with two different people. Then we try to get ourselves unsorted into a circle (or two joined circles) without letting go of anyone's hand.

Purpose: to demonstrate to the child that recovery untangles many problems in the family.

Journals – we write in our journals our personal plan to make healthy choices. What changes are we going to make, starting now? Who will we spend time with? Who are the safe people we will talk with to help us make healthy choices? How will we start to avoid risky situations? etc.

Purpose: to show the children it is not enough to just affirm we are going to make changes. We also need to make detailed plans.

Safe People – the parent asks the children who are the safe people in their lives, what makes them safe people, what qualities or characteristics do safe people tend to have in common, etc.

Purpose: children learn how to identify safe people for support and guidance.

Recovery Jeopardy – each child (or team) selects jeopardy questions from categories and gains points for correct answers. Jeopardy sheets for the game are included for recovery in the Supplemental materials at the end of this lesson.

Purpose: children learn many facts about recovery.

Meditation – we close our eyes and silently think of a scene of great beauty and peace (for a minute or two, depending on the age of the child). We imagine ourselves there. We notice everything around us. At the end we slowly open our eyes and take a few seconds to adjust back to our surroundings. At the end, we share our inner experience with others.

Purpose: to discover that peace is found inside us

Line in the Sand – put a long piece of masking tape along the floor, creating a tightrope. You have to work hard to keep your balance. Parent gently tosses soft toys at child, making it even more difficult. Parent asks children what these soft toys represent (life's difficulties). Ask the child to bend down and pick up a soft toy lying near the tape. Ask if this is difficult and what picking up the toy represents (extra effort that someone in early recovery must make to stay on the path to recovery).

Purpose: to understand life's challenges are to be met

with calm determination.

Journaling

Some suggested topics for this lesson are:

1. "One of my safe people is ___ and what makes her or him safe is _____ "

2. "I am going to take care of myself by ..."

3. Write a letter to recovery

Often, we give the child a choice of topics. When everyone is finished (including the parent), we may share what we have written.

Review – Treatment and Recovery

- Janie has made positive changes in her life. She has joined a 12-step group and no longer engages in self-destructive behaviors or uses drugs. We say that she has begun... what? (answer - her recovery)

- After several months of recovery, Jamie begins to slide back into old behaviors.   What is this called? (answer - relapse)

- For a while, Jamie makes excuses to herself and others for her changed attitudes and behaviors. She is engaging in ... what? (answer - denial)

- Finally, Janie admits to herself that spending time with her old using circle and skipping school and sneaking out late at night are not good for her. But she argues to herself that at least she hasn't started using drugs again, so everything's really okay. This is called ... what? (answer - more denial)

- Janie tells herself that she isn't relapsing because she's not using drugs. Is she right? (answer - no, relapse starts with going back to old thinking habits and old behaviors, and this usually happens well before one starts using drugs again)

- Finally, Janie starts using drugs again. She is arrested and the courts require her to get detoxed and go into treatment. While there, Jamie notices others whose drug habits are more advanced that hers. She tells herself, "At lease I'm not as bad as Bert or Andrea over there. I haven't gone to jail or lost my children." What is this kind of thinking called? (answer - more denial)

- Janie is told she is in "full-blown relapse". What does the term "full-blown relapse" mean? (answer - her relapse got to the point where she started to use drugs again)

- Even though she is back in treatment, Janie continues to use drugs. Then, she has a moment of clarity. She realizes she is in great danger. What should she do now? (answer - get back into recovery)

- Now Janie is serious again and is paying attention in her recovery group. Janie hears someone say, "Relapse is a part of recovery." Janie reacts angrily. "Are you saying it's okay to relapse?" she asks. What would you tell her? (answer - It's not okay to relapse. Relapse is extremely dangerous and if we do relapse we have to take responsibility for everything that happens. But relapse does happen to some people and when it does, it's important for them to get right back into recovery as quickly as possible.)

- Janie says, "I relapsed. Does that make me a bad person?" What would you tell her? (answer - no, it does not make you a bad person and you did well to get back into recovery. But you will need to make amends for any harm you caused.)

- Janie asks, "What does 'make amends' mean?" what would you tell her? (Making amends means you take responsibility for what you've done, you say you're sorry to the people you've hurt and you make a 'good faith' attempt to righting the wrongs, where possible)

Homework

- Do something fun and safe for yourself

OR

- Practice giving yourself an affirmation

The Seven C's

The Seven C's goes like this:

You didn't **C**ause it

You can't **C**ure it

You can't **C**ontrol it

But you **C**an take care of yourself, by

Making healthy **C**hoices for yourself

Communicating your feelings, and

Celebrating who you are

What I Liked Best About Today

Ask your child,

What did you like best about today?

Did you enjoy the time we spent together?

What is one important thing you learned today that you

didn't know before?

Serenity Pledge

Grant me the Serenity to accept the

people I cannot change,

The Courage to change the person I can,

And the Wisdom to know that person is me!

   - This ends today's lesson on Treatment

     and Recovery

Serenity Worksheet

Grant me the serenity to accept the things I cannot change

Here are some things I cannot change (in others):

1.

2.

3.

4.

5.

Courage to change the things I can

Here are some things I can change (in me):

1.

2.

3.

4.

5.

And the wisdom to know the difference

Here is a plan to take good care of me:

1.

2.

3.

4.

5.

Recovery

Recovery _feels_ like this: our teen girl begins a program of self-renewal with outside help (such as an AA 12-step program). She uses no alcohol or other drugs and begins to feel better physically. She also begins to experience her emotions more vividly. In the event of a relapse, she gets right back to her 12-step program with increased commitment, focus and humility.

Recovery _looks_ like this: our teenager learns to be completely honest with herself, makes amends to those she has wronged as far as she is able, and lets go of her shame. She learns to trust herself and others and gets in touch with all her feelings. She makes new friends in the recovery community and elsewhere. She learns to live again and finds that her life is getting better that it ever has been before. She begins to give back. She is an inspiration to others.

Signs of Relapse for a Person in Recovery

- Thinking difficulties
- Emotional overreactions
- Sleep disturbances
- Memory difficulties
- Becoming accident prone
- Experiencing serious sensitivity to stress
- Stopping communication
- Beginning to spend time convincing self/others everything is okay when it's not
- Avoiding people who give honest feedback
- Irritation/anger when given such feedback
- Everyday problems starting to become overwhelming, inability to solve them
- Feeling stuck/trapped/nowhere to turn
- Using magical thinking
- Becoming depressed
- Low energy
- Starting to think about suicide
- Impulsive behavior (thoughtless to self, others)
- Compulsive behavior – food, sex, caffeine, nicotine, work, gambling, etc.
- Urges and cravings for drugs
- Starting to use drugs again
- Refusal to take responsibility for starting again/justifications for continuing to use (oh, well, messed up, too late now, don't hold me responsible – I'm out of control so it's not my fault, I was born

to drink, may as well continue to use till I hit bottom, ...)

These are Dangerous for Relapse

- Exhaustion
- Dishonesty
- Impatience
- Need to be always right
- Depression
- Frustration
- Self-pity
- Boredom
- Being around using people, places and things
- Cockiness
- Complacency
- Unmet expectations of others
- Letting up disciplines
- Physical pain, unmanaged
- Unrealistic goals
- Forgetting gratitude
- Omnipotence / it can't happen to me

Skills for Relapse Prevention

or any other Impulsive Behavior Pattern

Signal – Stop – Question

- Signal – I am becoming aware I am about to be impulsive
- Stop – I need to stop and think about this
- What can I do

By using this technique, you will interrupt the impulsive thinking that might otherwise lead you to risky behavior. Be sure to focus on positive thoughts when following this process, such as:

- I really like staying safe
- I'm pleased with my progress so far in avoiding risky behavior
- I feel good when I work toward my goals

What are some of your ideas for positive thoughts like this?

Treatment and Recovery Jeopardy

- For 100 points: If someone becomes addicted, is the situation hopeless?

answer: no, recovery is always possible

- For 200 points: If a person relapses, does that mean the end of the person's recovery?

answer: no, as long as the person gets right back to the program with renewed purpose

- For 300 points: What are two powerful myths or misconceptions surrounding chemical dependency that people still believe today?

answer: that chemically dependent people are morally flawed and lacking in willpower

- for 400 points: What are two things we can do if someone we love is addicted and using?

answer: choose from: (a) stop enabling, (b) support loved one's efforts to recover, (c) arrange for a professional 'intervention' (if the family member won't admit problem and go for treatment), and (d) address our own recovery needs

- For 500 points: What is the difference between treatment and recovery?

answer: treatment addresses short-term medical and
   psychological needs.   It focuses on breaking the cycle
   of drug abuse.   Recovery is ongoing, living a different
   kind of life usually centered around the 12-step
   principles

- Daily Double: What are the Seven C's?

answer: I didn't cause it, I can't control it, I can't cure it -
   but I can take care of myself by making healthy
   choices, communicating my feelings and celebrating
   who I am.

Lesson Seven: Families

<u>Goals</u>:   Children learn …

1. that a family is a group of people who love each other
2. that all families are different
3. that no family is perfect
4. that all families are special
5. that all families have good times as well as problems and times of stress
6. that all families live with rules and that these rules are both spoken and unspoken, healthy and sometimes unhealthy (e.g., "We don't talk about that in this house." or "You don't really feel that way.")
7. the kinds of effects that addiction has on families

<u>Key Messages:</u>

All of us are part of a family. Our families may be very different. Some children may have two parents who live together while others may have parents who are divorced. Some of us may have other relatives who live with us, such as grandparents, aunts, uncles or cousins. Some of us may be adopted or live with foster parents. Some of us may be living with people who aren't actually related to us.

A family is any group of people who love each other and are involved with each other. Families provide love and support to one another. All families are different. All families are special. All families have good times as well as times of stress. In some families there is a lack of money. Some families may have someone with an illness or someone out of work. Some families may be homeless. There is no such thing as a perfect family.

Families are like teams. They work together, talk together, do different things together, and share things like living space, food, clothing, cars, etc. When a family works well together, talking and sharing are present. When not, and there is no talking nor sharing, there is often stress as well as other problems. However, even when a family might not be working well together, most parents and children love each other, and parents want to do the best they can for their children, and they do what they think is right.

When families are under stress, they often don't talk about how they feel or about their true problems. Sometimes they keep what's happening a secret from each other and from the outside world. Often family members blame each other for things that happen and hide their true feelings. Often the feeling of fear translates into anger or anxiety.

All families have rules. Some of the rules may be spelled out, talked about, maybe even written down. Many rules are implicit, that is, never discussed but picked up by the children from observing their parents and noticing how things work in their homes. Sometimes rules are confusing, because they are not clear or not consistently enforced. Usually when rules are confusing, children feel very insecure.

Everyone in a family has feelings. People don't always act the way they feel. Someone may act mad or angry with you, when the person is really worried about something else. Every family member has both strengths and weaknesses. Sometimes we don't notice all the likable, positive qualities about our family members. When someone is sick because of drugs or some other illness, we may see all the problems and forget the likable things about that person.

Our goal is to understand the impact in the family when there is a chemically dependent family member. A key point to recognize is that in families with addiction, members do not usually take regular care of themselves, that is self-care of emotions, feelings, needs, and overall health.

Alcoholism and other drug addictions cause people to act unpredictably, and often irrationally. You may not know what to expect from day to day. Since the other family members react to the addict's moods, they often become unpredictable, too. When someone in the family is chemically dependent, there may be more fighting, noise, broken promises, disappointments, misunderstandings, embarrassments, money problems, hidden feelings, physical and/or verbal abuse. Family members usually don't talk about the real issues or problems, and they keep what's happening in the family a secret. Chemical dependency is like a weight being put on a family member that throws the whole family out of balance.

Addiction is often found in some families in one

generation after another. This is due to genetic traits passed down from parent to child as well as a dysfunctional lifestyle that is passed down from one generation to the next. Recovery and education are the tools our society provides to help families break the addiction cycle.

Chemical dependency in a family has a great effect on everyone. In fact, it is called a "family disease" because everyone is so greatly affected. Families with chemical dependency often try to keep this secret from the rest of their extended family, their neighbors, their employers, their church, their school, and so on. This is sometimes called "the elephant in the living room". Children learn not to talk about the addiction to outsiders and often stop inviting friends over. The family may become very isolated. Fear, anger, shame and confusion can be an everyday fact of life.

There are lots of families in America dealing with addiction. It is estimated that between 20 and 28 million children live in a family affected with chemical dependency. Children with addiction in their families need to learn about their increased risk of developing chemical dependency themselves if they decide to use alcohol or other drugs. Their risk may be up to 4 times higher than the risks of their friends who do not have addiction in their families.

Children in families with addiction may experience a lot of loss. This could be loss of attention, loss of proper care, loss of opportunity to learn proper social skills and broken promises. They may feel fear, shame, anger, loneliness, disappointments and confusion. They often feel insecure and isolated. Because they may have to take on many responsibilities for their younger brothers and sisters, an older child may even feel the loss of his or her childhood. This is why all these family members and especially the children need to learn about addiction and its effect on families. They need to learn that their family's problems are not their fault and that they can find happiness and security by learning how to make healthy choices for themselves.

Please keep in mind that while all parents love their children, they don't always know how to show it or demonstrate responsible, encouraging and loving behaviors. Parents generally operate from their own experiences as children unless they have received help from others. Thus, poor parenting behaviors are often passed down from generation to generation in families with generational histories of addiction or other behavioral or psychological problems.

Activities

<u>Feelings Bag</u> – as described in Lesson Two (recommended for each lesson)

Purpose: children learn that we can ease the burden of uncomfortable feelings just by talking about them

<u>Draw a Picture of Your Family</u> – we draw a picture of our family showing each person. We add symbols such as a piano, hockey stick, newspaper, TV, etc. to show the interests of each family member. Then we share our pictures with the group.

Purpose: to show how our family fits together

<u>Journals</u> – we write in our journals " If I could change one thing about my family it would be…"

Purpose: to show the children that they have a voice in and vision for their family

<u>Play Dough</u> – we make play dough figures representing all the members of our family and share what the scene represents with others.

Purpose: to show the children every family is different and special

<u>Design a Wonderful Family</u> – use a whiteboard or poster board to brainstorm all the great qualities that a mother or father might have and another board to list all the great qualities children might have.

Purpose: for children to start thinking about how to improve how they relate to the world as part of a family, and to start thinking a little about what qualities they would like to develop by the time they are parents

Safe People – ask the children to think of as many safe people as they can and what kind of qualities these people have in common that make them safe. Be sensitive to children who indicate that they cannot think of a safe person. Suggest they think of a person who has played a significant role in their development.

Purpose: for children to start compiling their lists of safe people

Pillowcases – supply everyone with an inexpensive white pillowcase and colored fabric markers. Ask everyone to draw pictures of safe things on their pillowcases.

Purpose: children understand pillows are a safe place to rest our heads and our pillowcases protect our pillows, keeping them clean and safe from outside things like bugs and dirt. They symbolically represent protecting ourselves by making healthy choices so we reduce the likelihood of having negative consequences.

Journaling

Some suggested topics for this lesson are:

1. "If I could change one thing about my family it would be ..."

2. "I feel special when my family ..."

3. "What I add to my family is..."

Often, we give the child a choice of topics. When everyone is finished (including the parent), we may share what we have written.

Review – Families

- What makes a family a family? (answer – love and commitment)

- Is there a perfect family? (answer - no)

- Are all families okay? (answer – yes, as long as there is love and commitment. Some families are emotionally healthier than others.)

- Do families with alcohol and other drug dependencies have more problems? What kind? (answer – yes, in families with addiction, family members do not usually take regular care of themselves, that is self-care of emotions, feelings, needs, and overall health. There can also be legal and financial problems.)

- About how many children in America are living in a family affected by chemical dependency? (answer – between 20 and 28 million)

- Why would our genes affect our chances to become chemically dependent? (answer – statistics show a strong genetic component to the disease)

- How much more likely is a child with one chemically dependent parent to become chemically dependent him- or herself, compared to a friend who has no chemical dependency in her family? (up to four times more likely)

- How can we avoid becoming chemically dependent? (answer – the only sure way is to never start using)

- What needs is a family supposed to fulfill? (answer – love, involvement and emotional support)

- Do all families have rules? What are some example of family rules? (answer – they can be stated, such as Jimmie washes the dishes, Janie mows the lawn, Jerry takes out the trash, or unstated, such as we all sit down to dinner together, we treat each other with respect, and so on)

- Does chemical dependency affect the whole family? How? (answer – yes: fear, shame, anger, confusion, insecurity, ...)

- Why is a child in a family with chemical dependency more likely to become chemically dependent him- or herself? (answer – shared genes, stress, modeling of addictive behavior, emotionally unhealthy family environment, may have seen drugs being used, may have been offered drugs by a family member, unrelated users hanging around, etc.)

- Can chemical dependency skip a generation? (answer – yes, it often does, first because the genetic component can skip a generation, and secondly because unhealthy emotional patterns may be passed down from grandparents to a non-addicted parent, who nevertheless displays the same unhealthy emotional patterns, and then to the addicted child)

- Do all children in a family have the same chance to become chemically dependent? (answer – no, because while the family environment for all the children is roughly the same, the genetic components are only half shared between full siblings)

- How can we tell if we are going to become chemically dependent? (answer – we can't. None of us knows exactly how much alcohol or other chemical usage will tip us from use/abuse into addiction. Some people use alcohol in moderation their whole adult lives, for example, and only become alcoholics in their 60's or 70's.)

- What resources are available to children outside their families for help with chemical dependency? (answer – Alateen, school counselors, teachers, pastors or other religious leaders, and many more)

- Is chemical dependency called a 'family disease'? Why?   (answer – yes, because of the enormous impact it has on family functioning)

- Do you think a person can have 110 feelings a day?   (answer - yes)

Homework

- Name one thing you could do to make someone in your family feel loved and special. Now go home and do it!

- Parents, tell and show your children today that you love them.

The Seven C's

The Seven C's goes like this:

You didn't **C**ause it

You can't **C**ure it

You can't **C**ontrol it

But you **C**an take care of yourself, by

Making healthy **C**hoices for yourself

Communicating your feelings, and

Celebrating who you are

What I Liked Best About Today

Ask your child,

What did you like best about today?

Did you enjoy the time we spent together?

What is one important thing you learned today that you

   didn't know before?

Serenity Pledge

Grant me the Serenity to accept the

people I cannot change,

The Courage to change the person I can,

And the Wisdom to know that person is me!

- This ends today's lesson on Families

Family Matters

Families play an important part in our lives. Answer the following questions:

What makes a family a family?

What needs are families supposed to fulfill?

What one thing do you like best about your family?

What is one thing you would like to change in your family?

What do you add to your family?

Discussion Ideas

Do you think a child can cause his/her parents to drink or use other drugs?

Do you think a child can cause his/her parents to get divorced?

Do you think a child can get his/her divorced parents back together again?

Do you think a child's bad behavior, attitude or thoughts can cause a parent to get sick or become addicted?

Do you think if a child does 'everything right' it will solve problems in the family?

Do you think if a child loves a step-parent, guardian or foster parent, he/she is being disloyal to a birth parent?

Do you think that the more people who love a child the better it is for the child?

Do you think if a child gets angry with a parent who is relapsing, it will help push the parent back into recovery?

Do you think a child can change an adult's behavior?

Do you think it is okay to love a parent who is chemically dependent and using?   (it is okay; it is the only thing you can do for that person)

Family with Addiction

Self-Care Map

- The adult's job is to do treatment and recovery

- The kid's job is to do self-care (mind, body, feelings, spirit) and have fun (being a kid)!

Bubblegum Family Narrative

(Make a circle on the floor out of yarn)

We're going to do an activity now called the Bubblegum Family in order to show you what it looks like and feels like to live in a family with the disease of Chemical Dependency.

(Ask for volunteers to be Mom, Dad, Junior, and Sis)

Almost everyone has had an experience chewing bubblegum. Whether your favorite bubblegum is Hubba Bubba, Carefree, Bazooka or Bubble Yum bubblegum, there are all different kinds of bubblegum that people chew.

You know how someone can chew bubblegum for about 30 seconds and then take it out of his or her mouth? How does it feel? Sticky! It's really sticky and yucky. Here in the middle of the floor is an imaginary circle. We've stayed up the last 24 hours, and chewed piece after piece of bubblegum, all for 30 seconds. Then we've thrown each piece into the imaginary circle. Here in the circle are 9,997 pieces of slightly chewed bubblegum.

Here we have a family. *"Miss, please come up."* I want you to meet Mom. She is 35 years old, a mother of two, a wonderful mom. She has a full-time job that she is very good at. Just an incredible lady. She and her family are very happy. Since she's been a young adult, Mom has gone out each weekend drinking with her friends, but it doesn't seem to be a problem. All of a sudden as Mom is going through life, she steps right into the bubblegum. All of a sudden she's stuck. *"Try to move, Mom."* "Well, I'm trying but I can't really move much."

That's right, you can't move too much. That's addiction. People get stuck. Watch Mom. She can sway from side to side. She really thinks she's not stuck, that she can get out of that real quickly, but she can't. That's what DENIAL looks like! Denial is like telling yourself a lie.

What happens as time goes on is that Mom becomes more and more preoccupied with the gum while she's stuck in it. She can't do as good a job at work. She's out sick a lot. She can't be as productive because she's preoccupied with the gum. It's really starting to slow her down. She doesn't have freedom of choice anymore. When it comes to her kids, she can't take care of them like she used to. She's trapped in that gum, all the way up to her calf. She's stuck. She doesn't have as many choices as she had before. She's not spending as much time with her kids. Her kids can't count on her anymore to be there for them, to help them with homework or take them to after school activities. Or to bake their favorite chocolate chip cookies.

Mom has a husband called Dad. Dad loves his wife very much. Dad has been very concerned about Mom. *"Haven't you. Dad?"* "Why, yes.' Dad misses spending time with Mom. Dad has been concerned because he notices mom is stuck in the gum. She's on probation at work because she has been absent so many days. Her last work review wasn't very good. Dad has noticed over the last few months that he has had to take on more and more of the responsibilities at home. He's starting to prepare dinner most nights. He is also spending time helping the kids with their homework and helping them with their school projects on the weekend. He has even tried baking those chocolate chip cookies. He's very concerned about his wife. He doesn't get to spend much time with her alone because she seems preoccupied and distant. She's just stuck in that gum. He wants his life the way it used to be.

Because Dad loves Mom, what do you suppose he tries to do? He tries to free Mom from the bubblegum. *"So, go ahead, Dad, try to help Mom get out."*

As Dad tries to help Mom, all of a sudden he gets stuck in the bubblegum, too. Now he's stuck. *"Try to move around, Dad."* Notice he thinks he can move around and he thinks he's free, but he's really stuck. Remember that addiction is a progressive disease. When Mom first got stuck, the gum only went up to her calf. Now when Dad is stuck in there with her, it comes all the way up to just above her knees! So, how does this affect Dad? He is preoccupied at work. He's thinking about having to come home and prepare meals. He wonders if she's going to be drunk or sober. Will she embarrass him at the dinner party next week? He can't be as productive at work. He thinks more and more about her. He is not available to his kids on a consistent basis anymore. He doesn't always help them with their homework anymore.   So, all of a sudden he's stuck.   But, like Mom, he doesn't think he's stuck either.   For a long time, the family finds other reasons for their problems.   They make excuses and blame other people.

Now we have the older child, Junior.   Junior's very concerned because not only is Mom stuck but Dad's stuck, too.   Neither one is there for him on a consistent basis.   Now he's helping out his little sister with her homework, in addition to all his old chores.   He is having a hard time concentrating in school as he spends more and more time worrying and trying to make things work at home.   He doesn't always get his homework done. His grades are dropping. Junior doesn't have very many opportunities to play anymore because he's taking care of Sis.   He doesn't bring friends home anymore - he might get embarrassed by what's happening there.   When he does get a chance to play, he's often worried about Mom and Dad.   He might get yelled at for something he didn't do.

He's real concerned.   He misses his family the way it used to be.   He is going to try and get them unstuck. Now, Dad couldn't get Mom out of the pit.   Do you think Junior who is just a kid is going to be able to get them both out of the sticky bubblegum?   NO WAY!   He ends up stuck, too.   Now they are stuck up to their waists. Now, Sis wants her family back too and tries to get them unstuck.   Now the whole family is stuck up to their necks.

That's the Bubblegum Family.   Why do the kids get

stuck?   It's real important.   Why do the kids get stuck in the bubblegum?   They get stuck because they try to help their parents first.   So, if the reason why kids get stuck is because they try to help, how do kids get unstuck? Kids get unstuck when they stop trying to take care of other people in their families, like Mom, Dad, and brother and sisters.   They get unstuck when they begin to take good care of themselves.   That's how kids get unstuck from the bubblegum.

What does it mean to take care of yourself?   What are some different ways can kids take good care of themselves?   They can go out and play.   They can talk to a teacher.   Ask a counselor for help.   Go to a neighbor's house.   Call grandma if there's a mess at the house and you don't want to be there.   These are some of the different ways kids can take care of themselves.

Notice how everyone tried to help Mom.   They were all around her.   Everyone got stuck in the bubblegum.   Even if Mom wanted to get unstuck, she would have a hard time *because everyone is in the way*.   Each member of the family needs to get unstuck by him- or herself.   It begins by finding just one person you can trust and talk to and share your feelings with.   Sis's teacher notices she doesn't get along as well with the other children as she should.   She refers Sis to a social worker, who arranges for her to attend the a program at school.   Junior starts going to Alateen. Dad gets unstuck.   He goes to a new doctor who instead of writing a prescription for tranquilizers suggests he start going to Al Anon.   Dad starts going to Al Anon.

We have to remember that recovery takes time. There might be a time when Junior gets unstuck and starts to take good care of himself, but later Dad hosts a big dinner party at home for his business associates and Junior, trying to help out and handle more than he can, misses his Ala Teen meeting and doesn't get all his homework done. Afterwards, he sees what happened. *"Ah,"* he says to himself. *"I see what happened. Next time I'll let Dad know what I can't get done for him and let him figure out how to handle that while I make sure I get my homework done and my other needs met!"* Recovery is a process. We take two steps forward and, because we're human, sometimes we take a step backward. So we get stuck and unstuck, over and over again. But what happens over time is that when we start getting stuck we quickly become aware that we're getting stuck, so we don't stay stuck as long.

Now look what happens when everyone in the family is taking care of him- or herself and not trying to protect Mom. No one is blocking her path out of the pit to the road of recovery. She may finally see through the denial and realize that it is not her family that is causing all her problems. She is the one with the problem and she needs help. She can get unstuck by getting treatment or going to AA, or she might stay in the pit. It is her choice. Her family needs to stop trying to take care of her and instead, start taking care of themselves. This is not selfish. It is healthy for Dad and Junior and Sis. And it allows Mom a free path out of the pit when she is ready for it.

Effective Family Traits

1. Open to change and new ideas
2. Affirming; high-self worth
3. Conscious choice-making
4. Rules are designed to guide and protect; they are consistent and appropriate
5. Feelings are expressed openly and validated ("I understand you are feeling ...")
6. Sense of safety and security; touch and communications are appropriate and nurturing
7. Stress is usually anticipated and dealt with directly and effectively; family members pull together for mutual support
8. Parents are in charge – a strong coalition using clear, direct communication
9. Fun, humor, laughter and joy are valued, encouraged and enjoyed
10. Life-stages are accepted and age-appropriate rules and expectations are set; parents are parents and children are children
11. Personal and holiday celebrations/ acknowledgments occur regularly, reliably and dependably

Ineffective Family Traits

1. Rigid, black-and-white thinking
2. Shame-based, low self-worth
3. Compulsive behaviors
4. Arbitrary, rigid or non-existent rules
5. Feelings are avoided and repressed (except possibly anger and rage)
6. No sense of safety; there are risks from others to mind, body and spirit
7. Denial of stress, issues and problems   OR stress is a welcome distraction from one's own emotional pain
8. Disturbed hierarchy: either one person dominates the family   OR   nobody is in charge; hidden coalitions; "upside –down" family structure; chaotic, crisis-mode functioning
9. Terminal seriousness: rarely happy, upbeat or optimistic; usually depressed, angry or hostile OR   phony happiness (everything's FINE)
10. Disturbed developmental process resulting in either "the eternal toddler"   OR   "the parenting child"
11. Passage of time is ignored: lack of or limited acknowledgment of birthdays, anniversaries, holidays, bar/bat mitzvahs, confirmations, school and work accomplishments

Family Values

a. Honesty
b. Integrity
c. Compassion

d. Decency/modesty
e. Kindness
f. Mercy

g. Charity
h. Humility
i. Hygiene/self-care

j. Loyalty
k. Tolerance
l. Sobriety

m. Fortitude/courage
n. Faithfulness

Family Values Worksheet

Put the letter of the Family Value next to each statement below:

John gave Sam a copy of the answers to the biology test. Sam tore it up without looking at it and took the test using his own brainpower. This Family Value is: (answer: b. – Integrity)

Kerry's brother was worried that their dad wouldn't come to pick them up after school. But Kerry was sure their dad would come. This Family Value is: (answer: n. – Faithfulness)

James saw that Sarah was short by $5.00 to pay for her groceries and she was really embarrassed in the checkout line. He offered to help her by lending her the $5.00. This Family Value is: (answer: e. – Kindness)

Sarah found a wallet on the ground. She was able to find the owner's name and address, so she mailed it back to him. She didn't take any of the wallet's contents. This Family Value is: (answer: a. – Honesty)

Tim saw a homeless man shivering in the cold. He bought him a cup of hot cocoa and offered him his coat. This Family Value is: (answer: c. – Compassion)

Mark borrowed his friend Robert's car. He was driving carelessly and wrecked the car. Mark felt terrible and asked Robert to forgive him for being so careless. Robert forgave his friend. This Family Value is: (answer: f. – Mercy)

Sarah couldn't afford to give to the poor, so she worked at the Soup Kitchen once a month to help others less fortunate than herself. This Family Value is: (answer: g. – Charity)

When Gary's car broke down, he decided to walk the rest of the way to work instead of giving up. This Family Value is: (answer: m – Fortitude/courage)

Barry got the highest score on a test. He didn't boast to his classmates because he didn't want to make them feel less important. This Family Value is: (answer: h. – Humility)

Though all of Kim's friends were going to a party where there would be drinking and pot smoking, Kim decided to stay home and give herself a facial, pedicure and manicure. This Family Value is: (answer: l. – Sobriety)

At a sleepover, the girls were gossiping about Carol who wasn't at the party. Carol's friend Jane asked the others to stop talking about Carol because it made her feel uncomfortable to talk about her friend Carol behind her back. This Family Value is: (answer: j. – Loyalty)

Jerry saw a group of Muslims praying together before boarding the same airplane he was flying. Jerry respected the group and passed buy without making any comment or gesture. This Family Value is: (answer: k. – Tolerance)

Karen saw two skirts she really liked while shopping. One was really cute but extremely short. The other was also really cute, but a little longer, and not as provocative. Karen chose the longer one. This Family Value is: (answer: d. – Decency/Modesty)

Mary takes a shower, brushes her teeth and styles her hair every day. She wants to look her best and smell clean. This Family Value is: (answer: i. – Hygiene/Self-Care)

Positive Traits and their Opposites

Live the Values You Admire – Do it Today!

Polite   (*not* – rude)

Humorous and Fun-loving   (*not* –   stoic, humorless, straight-faced)

Forthright–honest about feelings and motivations (*versus* – manipulative)

Reliable   (*not* – unpredictable)

Hard-working   (*not* – unmotivated)

Mentally-engaged   (*not* – foolish, unprepared)

Peace-loving and non-violent   (*not* – violent, aggressive)

Self-reliant   (*not* – dependent)

Integrity and honesty   (*not* – sneakiness, deceitfulness)

Sobriety   (*not* – drunk, high, buzzed)

Fortitude and courage   (*not* – defeatist, cowardice)

Trusting   (*not* – suspicious, prying)

Humble   (*not* – bragging, boasting)

Loyal   (*not* – untrustworthy, betraying)

Compassionate   (*not* – indifferent)

Merciful   (*not* – unforgiving)

Decent and modest   (*not* – indecent, provocative, immoral)

Tolerant and understanding   (*not* – critical, judgmental, intolerant)

Kind   (*not*–cruel)

Generous and charitable   (*not* – stingy, greedy)

Cooperative and democratic   (*not* – domineering, stubborn)

Hygienic and self-caring   (*not* – unclean, messy, dirty)

Physically Fit   (*not* – unhealthy, unfit, self-damaging)

Faithful and spiritual   (*not* – fearful and confined)

Hopeful   (*not* – despairing)

Lesson Eight: Peer Pressure and Decision Making

<u>Goals:</u>   Children ...

1. learn that all of us, even adults, are faced with peer pressure sometimes
2. learn that we all make decisions every day
3. learn that we are all responsible for our own choices
4. learn how to think about choice and consequences
5. practice making a healthy/safe decision
6. practice refusal skills - saying "No"

<u>Key Messages:</u>

Peers are our equals, that is our friends, neighbors, schoolmates and so on. Because people are social creatures, we feel a need to belong to a group and a pressure to conform to our group's expectations. This is called *peer pressure*. Everyone is subject to peer pressure, even adults. Peer pressure can be healthy or unhealthy. Healthy peer pressure might be a schoolmate asking you to study with her for tomorrow's big history test, or a teammate asking you to practice basketball with him on the weekend before a big game coming up.

Unhealthy peer pressure is when our friends urge us to do something that we know is not right for us. It might be to skip school, to shoplift, to have sex, to cheat on a test, and so on. One unhealthy peer pressure is when our friends urge us to try alcohol or other drugs. The pressure can be casual (hey, you want some...) or more overt (come on, don't be a chicken...). The pressure might not even be anything our friends do or say, just a desire in our own head to 'fit in' (well, they're all drinking, I guess I'll have some ...).

We all make decisions every day, such as what we will wear and what we will eat. It is important that we know how to make healthy and safe choices. That takes thinking about options and possible consequences. When we are very young, our parents make most decisions for us. As we get older, we are allowed to make more decisions for ourselves. This means the child must stop and think about options, possible consequences and which option helps him/her to move closer to his/her goals.

One of parents' main jobs is to transition responsibility for specific decision making to a child as soon as the child is safely able to take on the particular responsibility. For example, at an appropriate age, a parent should transition responsibility for waking up on time and doing school assignments to the child.

It is important to remember that everyone is responsible for the decisions one makes. That means we accept responsibility for our choices and deal with the consequences. People who are chemically dependent and abusing drugs usually do not take responsibility for their decisions and actions unless they are forced to. Often it is a consequence imposed from outside that brings a drug abuser to treatment. That consequence can be legal, or a job loss, or divorce, or the loss of a home, etc. The consequence can also be imposed by a family member who decides not to enable the user any longer, that is, not to clean up after him/her, lie or make excuses - in short, no longer to shield the person from the consequences of using.

The STAR model helps us make effective decisions and implement them. The 'S'stands for Stop, meaning stop and consider what alternatives are available. The 'T' means to think of all the things I need to do to make this work. The 'A' stands for Act, to act decisively and with respect to all concerned. And the 'R'stands for Review, which means to check out how the action worked, whether it needs to be repeated or modified, and how we feel about the results.

Activities

<u>Feelings Bag</u> – as described in Lesson Two (recommended for each lesson)

Purpose: children learn that we can ease the burden of uncomfortable feelings by talking about them

<u>Journals</u> – each child writes about a time he or she didn't yield to peer pressure.

Purpose: children learn that it is okay to say "no"

<u>How to Say "No" and Keep Your Friends</u> – children use m&m's to practice how to say "no" and keep their friends. Be sure to tell the children before the exercise starts that the candy is just candy, and does not represent drugs. One child (or a parent if only one child is present) asks another to try the m&m's. The pressuring person uses all the skills, reasons and persuasive powers that come to mind to convince the child to eat an m&m. The child being tempted uses the Refusal Chart (find chart in the Supplemental materials at the end of the lesson) to formulate a refusal that makes sense based on what temptation language was used. The one doing the tempting puts ever more pressure on the refusing child. The refusing child uses ever more firm refusals from the chart to say "no." When everyone has had the chance to be the one tempting and the one refusing, the children may be allowed to eat their m&m's. (parent's choice)

Purpose: children practice using refusal skills and learn

there are many ways to refuse to do things they feel pressured to do

Tear Yourself Away– children experience the difficulty of "tearing away" from peer pressure by joining in a paper-tearing game. Give each child 3 pieces of paper and a pencil. Say, "Sometimes our friends pressure us to do things we don't really want to do. If only one or two people pressure us it may be easy to say 'no.' But when everyone pressures us together, it's hard not to give in. On the first piece of paper write something your friends have pressured you to do. Now fold the paper in half. Pretend the fold represents one person pressuring you, saying "Do it. No one will ever know!" Now tear your paper in two. Was it easy to do? Is it hard to say 'no' to just one person? Why or why not? Repeat the process with the next piece of paper, but this time have the child fold it over twice, representing two peers pressuring. Ask, "Was it a little harder to tear the paper this time?" Finally, do the same with the third piece of paper, but ask the children this time to fold it over five times. Repeat the questions, noting how the paper become increasing hard to tear the more times it's folded. Ask, "How do the folds in this paper act like peer pressure? Why is it harder to say 'no' to several friends than it is to say 'no' to just one?

Purpose: children learn it's harder to resist peer pressure when more people are applying it together

Journaling

Some suggested topics for this lesson are:

1. "One time I didn't yield to peer pressure was ..."

2. "The times I feel most pressured are ..."

3. "My best way to say 'no' is..." (clarification, if

   required: best = most effective)

4. "Some of the problems teenagers face today are ..."

Often, we give the child a choice of topics. When everyone is finished, including parent(s), we may share what we have written.

Review – Peer Pressure

- What is "peer pressure"? (answer – pressure that is put on you by others your age)

- Is "peer pressure" always negative or bad? (answer – no)

- What are some kinds of "positive peer pressure"? (answer – a friend calls you to ask if you want to study for the test together, a friend calls to ask if you want to play some basketball, a friend calls to ask you to the movies,...)

- What are some examples of "negative peer pressure"? (answer – a friend asks to copy your homework, a friend asks you to give her the answers during the biology test, a schoolmate offers you alcohol or another drug,...)

- Is it possible to say "no" and still keep your friends? (answer – yes, and sometimes we gain respect and social points by standing up for ourselves)

- What are some of the ways we practiced "saying no"? (answer – see sheet in Supplemental materials at the end of the chapter)

Review – Decision Making

- What are some examples of decisions we make every day? (answer – what to wear, what to eat, whether to do our homework, what to do after school, ...)
- Are we all responsible for our own choices? (answer – yes)
- What does it mean to be responsible for a choice we have made? (answer – it means we accept responsibility for the choice and deal with the consequences)
- Do people who are chemically dependent, and using, take responsibility for their choices? (answer – no, unless forced to)
- If a person "cleans up" after a person who is abusing alcohol or other drugs, what is that called? (answer – enabling)
- Is someone who is enabling making healthy choices for him- or herself? (answer – no, we hurt ourselves while not really helping the person we are trying to help)
- What is something we can do to *really* help someone who is abusing alcohol or other drugs? (answer – *stop enabling*, and start taking care of ourselves)
- Is that always easy to do if one is a child or a teen, and the one abusing is a parent? (answer – no, not at first. But it gets easier the longer the child/teen

practices the Seven C's)

- What do the 'S' 'T' 'A' and 'R'   in the STAR Problem Solving Model stand for? (answer – **S**top, **T**hink, **A**ct and **R**eview)
- What was the problem we worked using the STAR model? Do you remember?

Homework

- (If 'Tear Yourself Away' activity was covered)

  Participants write on a piece of paper the name of a safe person or the name of a parent, then folds the paper over several times. Taking the paper back to their room that night they unfold the paper, read the name, and reflect how a person's love is stronger that peer pressure

- Practice ways to say, "no"

The Seven C's

The Seven C's goes like this:

You didn't **C**ause it

You can't **C**ure it

You can't **C**ontrol it

But you **C**an take care of yourself, by

Making healthy **C**hoices for yourself

Communicating your feelings, and

Celebrating who you are

What I Liked Best About Today

Ask your child,

What did you like best about today?

Did you enjoy the time we spent together?

What is one important thing you learned today that you

    didn't know before?

Serenity Pledge

Grant me the Serenity to accept the

people I cannot change,

The Courage to change the person I can,

And the Wisdom to know that person is me!

- This ends today's lesson on Peer
Pressure and Decision Making

How to Say 'No' and Keep Your Friends

- Have a Better Idea

- Make an Excuse

- Change the Subject

- Ignore it

- Act Shocked

- Say – No, Thanks

- Say – I don't want to!

- Say <u>Firmly</u> - No, that's **NOT** for me!

- **Leave** (without saying anything)

Note: refusals become **more adamant** the further down the list one goes

Peer Pressure Quiz

- What kind of pressure might your friends put on you? List some.
  (*answers*: (a) threats of isolation from the group, e.g., cold shoulders, (b) being excluded from group activities, (c) losing a boyfriend or girlfriend, (d) put-downs, teasing, (e) threats of bodily harm, (f) manipulation through guilt and shame (someone implies that if you won't do something they ask of you, that you don't love or care about them, or you are not a true friend, or that you are a bad person)

- What can you do about peer pressure? List some things.
  (*answers*: (a) Stop and Think about what is the best choice considering options and consequences, (b) remember that peers may use "roadblocks" of manipulation and children need to learn to take "detours" to stay on the right track, (c) remember if someone is using alcohol or other drugs, that person cannot be reasoned with, and there is no purpose in having a discussion with that person until he/she is sober)

- Violence Impact – sometimes people become angry and verbally or physically abusive when you refuse to do what they ask. This is especially true if the person has been using drugs. It is best to take care of yourself and use a safe person if necessary. Also, some people are by nature abusive personalities (see chart 'Signs of an Abuser' in the Supplemental materials at the end of the **next** chapter). What should one do when encountering an abusive person?

(*answer*: It is best to get away from that person immediately and use a safe person to prevent further contact, if necessary)

STAR Problem Solving Model

Stop –   What is the problem? Name it.

Remember: you don't need to do what you have always done before , especially if it didn't work.

Remember: you don't need to react to an uncomfortable feeling you might be having just now.

Think –   How do I feel? How can I solve this problem? What are my options? Do I need the help of others or some other resources? Which options help me stay safe and allow me to take good care of myself?

Remember: you can always ask others you respect for their help or opinions.

Act –   Act decisively with respect to all concerned.

Remember: I can take care of myself.

Remember: I can make healthy choices.

Review –   How do I feel? Did I get the result I expected? Did I get the result that deep down I really wanted? Did this action work for me? Would I try to solve this problem or a similar one the same way again? What might I do differently next time? Do I want to tell somebody what I've accomplished?

Remember: I can communicate my feelings.

Remember: I can celebrate who I am and what I've accomplished.

REMEMBER: A Good Choice Keeps Me Safe While Advancing Me Toward My Goals

Wheel of Misfortune
Use the STAR Method to Address these Situations in Small Groups

Pick and choose from among the following or make up your own:

a. A girl is blamed unfairly by her teacher …

b. A boy is yelled at for no reason by his mother …

c. A girl's best friend passes out at a party …

d. A girl's father comes by after school to pick her up, but he's drunk …

e. A young boy's single mother has not come home and it's 2:30 a.m. …

f. A girl's father is beating up her mother …

g. A boy's best friend asks him to come over after school to drink beer …

h. A girl is with her best friends when another girl comes by and tells her she has a food stain on her clothes

i. A boy's dad and mom are angry with each other

and not talking. When his mother has something to say to his dad, she tells her son to tell the father ...

j.   A girl's younger brother is being hit by her father ...

k.   A boy's father has promised to take him fishing, but now says he never promised ...

l.   A girl's father and mother are getting divorced, but nobody's said so to her ...

m.   A boy's friend has started shoplifting ...

n.   A girl finds empty beer cans in her teen brother's closet ...

o.   A girl's older brother hurt her physically when he got mad ...

p.   A boy's mom left him alone all weekend while she went out drinking ...

q.   A boy's friends are teasing a kid who is different and they want him to join in ...

r.   A boy's sister keeps coming into his room ...

s.   A boy's mom wants him to come live with her. He doesn't want to hurt her feelings, but he wants to stay with his dad ...

t. A new friend asks a girl to come over and she agrees. Then the girl's best friend calls and asks her to come over at the same time and she would rather be with her best friend …

u. A boy's not sick but he doesn't feel well …

v. A girl's big sister destroys her property, then blames it on her …

w. A boy's babysitter is drinking and doesn't want him to tell his parents …

x. A group of girls is always threatening a girl in the bathroom at school …

y. A boy and a girl got left in their car for a long while while their dad was in a bar …

z. A girl sitting next to a boy in math class wants to see his answers on the test they are taking …

Using the STAR Decision-Making Method

Whenever you're faced with making a decision, it's important to consider many alternatives. One way to determine these alternatives is to ask a lot of different people what they would do. Read over the example done for you below.

Which idea under 'THINK (FIRST)' appeals to you the most? Circle your choice. Did you consider the risks/consequences for each alternative?

STOP: State the Situation

Jan has to make a decision about going to a show on the night before a big biology test. She wants to see the show with her friends, but she should study for the test in order to get a good grade.

THINK (FIRST): Feelings, Ideas (and consequences), Resources, Safety, Take care of me

- *First Idea & Consequences*

Go to the show and don't worry about studying for the test. Ask your child: what are the possible consequences? *(answer - Flunk the test. Have fun - or might not have fun if worrying about my choice).*

- *Second Idea & Consequences*

Don't go to the show. School grades are more important. Ask your child: what are the possible consequences? *(answer - Prepare for test, and feel good about going to* school the next day, but feel resentful that I never get to do anything fun.)

- *Third Idea & Consequences*

Ask the teacher to postpone the test because so many kids want to see the show. Ask your child: what are the possible consequences? *(answer* - Teacher might say yes. Teacher might say no. It may be too late to try this idea.)

- *Fourth Idea & Consequences*

Study for the test before and after the show, but go to the show. Ask your child: what are the possible consequences? *(answer* - Prepare for test. Feel good about going to school the next day. Also feel good about treating myself to a fun activity.)

ACTION: My choice

Prioritize the ideas to select the action I want to take. Then take the action feeling confident that my choice is safe and takes good care of ME, and that I can live with the consequences that might follow.

REVIEW: Result

Think about what happened as a result of the decision I made and the action I took. Did I keep myself safe? Did I take good care of my future and myself? How do I feel about my decision now? How would I handle this situation if it happens again?

What Influences My Decisions?

The people and things around you influence the decisions you make. For example, your parents affect your actions, but so do the TV shows you watch and the attitudes of friends and others you respect. Below, make two lists of the people and things that influence you the most. If possible, rank them in order of importance, with the most important at the top.

Here are the people who influence me:

Here are the things that influence me:

Answer and discuss:

Do I feel comfortable with the top influences in both categories?   Why or why not?

Which influences would I like to change, or reduce in importance?

Which influences will change as I get older?

What influences my decisions about whether to use alcohol or other drugs? Explain.

Healthy Decisions

Your choices in life, especially ones that involve really important matters, shape your future and may determine your destiny. You can influence your future in positive ways by learning to make good decisions. The exercises below are designed to help you understand:

- How decisions that you face every day are important in determining your future
- The people and things that influence your decisions, and
- The steps to take to make good decisions.

How important are my decisions?
Everyone makes decisions daily. Some of the decisions are more important than others. Some are so important that they require thought, much study, and investigation before a wise decision can be made. Others are simply automatic. Here are some kinds of decisions that affect you:

A) Decisions not under your control, that is, those made by others
B) Automatic decisions, the ones you don't think about before acting
C) Decisions you occasionally think about beforehand
D) Decisions you think about but don't study or investigate beforehand
E) Decisions you study, think about a little, and ask others about before deciding

F) Decisions you study and think about a lot before deciding. You ask others questions and consider their answers before deciding.

Directions: The following list of 14 decisions is typically faced by most people.   How would you make each of them? Use the code letters (A B C D E F) to assess these decisions. If a particular decision isn't appropriate for you, leave it blank.

Decisions I make:
To get up in the morning
To tell the truth
To criticize a friend behind his or her back
To take a summer job
What to eat and when
To do my homework
To go to school
What movie to see
To use alcohol or other drugs
Where to dispose of waste paper
To report cheating to the teacher
To stop at a stop sign
What musical instrument to take up
To smoke cigarettes

Lesson Nine: Self Care and Getting Help

<u>Goals:</u> Children learn …

1. that there are many areas of their lives that require self care
2. that it is okay to ask a safe person for help
3. how to get help

<u>Key Messages:</u>

As we get older we all take on more of the responsibility for taking care of ourselves. When we were babies, our parents did everything for us. As we become adults, we take on the full responsibility for our care. Self care involves taking care of our bodies, our minds, our spirits, our feelings, our social needs and our goals and hopes. It means that we are responsible for our own happiness.

In order to take care of ourselves we need to know what rights we have as teens. These include the right to be treated with respect, the right to say 'no' to inappropriate touch, drugs, or negative behavior, the right to have our own feelings, opinions and beliefs, the right to get angry, the right to make mistakes, the right to change our mind, the right to not take responsibility for anyone else's negative behavior, and the right to ask for help and emotional support.

It's important for all of us to have safe people around us whom we trust and who we know love us. We want always to have someone available to us with whom we can share our joys and sorrows, our successes and misfortunes, and to whom we can turn for advice and support during difficult times.

Activities

Feelings Bag – as described in Lesson Two (recommended for each lesson)

Purpose: children learn that we can ease the burden of uncomfortable feelings by talking about them

Journals – parents and children write **about a time when they asked for help.**

Purpose: children learn that it is a good thing to ask for help when it is needed

Self-Care Jeopardy – children select questions and compete with each other to gain the most points for correct answers.

Purpose: to talk about self-care in a game format

Safe People Characteristics – children brainstorm what qualities a safe person is going to have and these are written down on a chart or white board. The children are asked to think about who the safe people in their lives are, and make a written list. At the end the parent can sum up as follows: "We've been talking about safe people and safe places. We know how important it is to share our feelings instead of holding them inside where they can do us harm. But we can't share our feelings with everyone, can we? We've also learned that we can get help with our problems, but we have to ask for it. However, there are some people we really can't ask, right. We need to have safe people we can talk to or call on when we need help. We also need to have safe places to go when we are feeling uncomfortable or unsafe."

Purpose: children begin to understand that safe people have a common set of characteristics and identify who is safe for them right now

Positive Messages – (for three or more children) each participant gets a piece of colored paper and writes his or her name at the top. Then the papers are passed around to all participants, including parents, and everybody writes something special and positive about the person whose name is at the top of the paper. When the papers finally arrive back at the originating child, he or she reads the messages aloud to the group.

Purpose: to understand the importance of receiving positive messages and affirmations from others, both other children and adults

Water Balloon Toss – (warm weather only) each participant picks a partner and the partners get a balloon filled with water. Outside, we begin tossing our balloon gently back and forth, trying to keep it from breaking while gradually increasing the distance between us.

Purpose: this reinforces the concept of safe person being there for us, even though the safe person may grow distant at some time in life

Wastebasket – all participants line up behind one another

and the first in line gets a wadded up piece of paper. The participant is asked a question and if she/he gets the answer right one point is scored. (Ideally the questions should be 'slam dunks' so everyone feels good about what each has learned.) Then the person tries to make a "basket" by throwing the paper wad into the basket, for a second chance to score a point. Participants keep track of their own points and the game is played for between two and five rounds, depending on the size of the group. Children report back to the group how many points they have scored and may get prizes in addition to recognition. (parent discretion)

Purpose: another learning opportunity in a fun setting

Sticks and Stones – make a chart or on a white board list two headings: (1) positive things I would like people to say about me, and (2) negative things that I don't want people to say about me. Start the exercise by stating, "Sticks and stones may break my bones, but words will never hurt me!" Ask the participants if they believe that statement. Most kids will say they don't believe it, that some of the worst pain comes from verbal abuse and mean words.

Ask participants to brainstorm according to the two chart headings. Afterwards, read through all the negative statements (without referring to anyone at all) and ask the children how they felt hearing those things even when they were not directed at them. Do the same for the positive statements and ask how they felt hearing those words. Assure them they are unique and special and tell them they need to hold on to positive statements to counteract negative messages we all get from time to time.

Purpose: for children to learn the power of words

<u>Self-Care Analysis</u> – What does "grant me the wisdom to accept the people I cannot change" mean for us? If we can't change them, what can we do about the behavior that is adversely affecting us? Talk to them about using "I" messages, that state how we are feeling about a behavior, and that can't be challenged because only we know how we feel. Counsel them that we can always talk to a safe person about the behavior and ask for help if we feel the behavior is putting us in danger. Advise that we can also leave the room, write about our feelings in a journal, etc.

What does "… and the wisdom to know that person is me" mean? What can we change about ourselves? (outlook, attitude, reactions)

Purpose: we will focus today on things we can do to change ourselves, protect ourselves and take care of ourselves. When you were a small child, your parents were responsible to take care of you. Some parents, especially those who are either chemically dependent or focused on someone else in the family who is, just aren't able to take care of children the way they might otherwise. We don't have to judge these parents as bad or unworthy. We can learn to accept them as they are. We don't have to accept their unacceptable behavior, but we can try to love them as they are, and take care of ourselves as best we are able in their spiritual absence.

Journaling

Some suggested topics for this lesson are:

1. "One time I asked for help was ..."

2. "One way I take good care of myself is ..."

3. "Something I need help with right now is ..."

4. What does shame look like to you? (write a poem, rap song, draw a picture, ...)

5. "One thing I get blamed for that's not my fault is ..."

6. "One time I stood up for myself was ..."

Often, we give the child a choice of topics. When everyone is finished (including the parent), we may share what we have written.

Review – Self Care and Getting Help

- What are some of the important parts of ourselves that we need to take care of? (answer – our minds, our bodies, our feelings, our spirit and our social needs)

- Is it all right to ask for help when we need it? (answer – yes)

- To whom should we go for help? (answer – a safe person whom we trust and who we think will have the knowledge and commitment to help us)

- Do children have rights? (answer – many rights, and, children, please do get familiar with your Bill of Rights)

- Do parents have rights? (answer – yes, the same ones)

The Seven C's

The Seven C's goes like this:

You didn't **C**ause it

You can't **C**ure it

You can't **C**ontrol it

But you **C**an take care of yourself, by

Making healthy **C**hoices for yourself

Communicating your feelings, and

Celebrating who you are

What I Liked Best About Today

Ask your child,

What did you like best about today?

Did you enjoy the time we spent together?

What is one important thing you learned today that you

didn't know before?

Serenity Pledge

Grant me the <u>Serenity</u> to accept the

people I cannot change,

The <u>Courage</u> to change the person I can,

And the <u>Wisdom</u> to know that person is me!

- This ends today's lesson on Self Care
and Getting Help

Serenity Worksheet

Grant me the serenity to accept the things I cannot change

Here are some things I cannot change (in others):

1.

2.

3.

4.

5.

Courage to change the things I can

Here are some things I can change (in me):

1.

2.

3.

4.

5.

And the wisdom to know the difference

Here is a plan to take good care of me:

1.

2.

3.

4.

5.

Children's Personal Bill of Rights
(these are for parents, too!)

- I have the right to be treated with respect

- I have the right to say "No" to inappropriate touch, drugs, and negative behavior

- I have the right to have my own feelings, opinions, and beliefs

- I have the right to get angry

- I have the right to make mistakes

- I have the right to change my mind

- I have the right to not take responsibility for anyone else's problems or negative behavior

- I have the right to ask for help and emotional support

Now, let's talk about these rights ...

- Do I have the right to dream big?

- Do I have the right to support and encouragement from those who love me?

- Do I deserve to be happy?

- Do I have the right to make my own decisions? Why or why not?

- Do I have the right to do whatever I want? Why or why not?

Self-Care

My Happiness depends on taking care of my mind, my body, my social needs (being a kid), my spirit, my feelings, and having goals and hopes (thinking big!)

A Personal Guide for Living

Many people find it helpful to develop a personal guide for living. Such a document is meant to be dynamic, changing as one uses it and experiences new things. Here as an example is my guide, today:

1. I live in the present moment

2. I look inside for happiness

3. I look outside for engagement (with the world)

4. I love myself just as I am now and as I always was

5. I let all anger go

6. I forgive myself for all my mistakes and for my personal shortcomings

7. I affirm that I've always done the best I could

8. I accept my failures and learn from them

9. I am honest about harm I do to others and sincere in my apologies

10. I accept that one who harms me does so because his/her heart is not yet capable of seeing and loving

11. I learn compassion by forgiving

12. I abide in the question, open to dialogue and change

13. I compare myself to no one (neither to satisfy my ego

nor to stand in judgment)

14. Feeling stuck, I look outside myself by starting a project, a relationship, a conversation or seeing the beauty around me

15. I ask for what I need and work with what is offered

Self-Care Jeopardy – Mind

- For 100 points: What are five things we can do to improve our minds?

answer: examples are read, go to a museum, write a poem, talk to someone older and wiser, learn to play chess, learn another language, etc.

- For 200 points: What are two mood-altering drugs? (hint: these are both legal for adults)

answer: caffeine and nicotine

- For 300 points: What are five mind-altering drugs? (hint: a person in recovery can never use any of these drugs without relapsing)

answer: cocaine, marijuana, LSD, heroin, alcohol, prescription pain pills, speed, peyote, meth, etc.

- for 400 points: What organ of the body do alcohol and other mind-altering drugs affect almost immediately?

answer: the brain

- For 500 points: True or False, someone else can make me mad?

answer: false. Our emotions come from inside us, not from outside

- Daily Double: What are the Seven C's?

answer: I didn't cause it, I can't control it, I can't cure it - but I can take care of myself by making healthy choices, communicating my feelings and celebrating who I am.

Self-Care Jeopardy – Body

- For 100 points: How many hours of sleep does the average person need each night?

answer: seven to eight, but children and teenagers need an hour or two more

- For 200 points: Name two reasons it is not right for professional athletes to use steroids

answer: negative effect on personal health, the image of their sport, negative effect on young fans, and others

- For 300 points: What are three things we do every day for good personal hygiene?

answer: bath/shower, brush teeth, brush hair, floss, use deodorant, dress in clean clothes, etc.

- for 400 points: Name two healthy ways a person can get stronger?

answer: eat right and exercise

- For 500 points: Name two ways, one for tobacco and one for alcohol, that a person can die as a result of another person's use?

answer: second-hand smoke and car crash

- Daily Double: At what age is a young person's brain fully developed?

answer: about age 26

Self-Care Jeopardy – Feelings

- For 100 points: Name three feelings that might cause a young person to experiment with alcohol or other drugs?

answer: curiosity, boredom, depression (among many others)

- For 200 points: Are feelings good or bad? Or, is it better to say, 'Feelings just are'

answer: feelings just are, and it's how we handle them that counts

- For 300 points: What do we use when we want to hide our true feelings?

answer: defenses

- for 400 points: What are three things people should never do when they have uncomfortable feelings?

answer: hurt themselves or others, or break things

- For 500 points: What are four healthy ways to handle uncomfortable feelings?

answer: talk, meditate, journal, exercise, deep breathing, …

- Daily Double: Name the feeling that usually has other feelings hiding behind it?

answer: anger, that sometimes hides fear,

embarrassment, hurt, worry, jealousy, etc.

Self-Care Jeopardy – Spirit

- For 100 points: What are some places that some people sometimes go to renew their spiritual needs?

answer: church, temple, synagogue, mosque, meditation retreat

- For 200 points: What does a pep rally at school attempt to generate?

answer: school spirit

- For 300 points: What does it mean when people say someone is "high spirited"?

answer: lively, playful, energetic, joyful

- for 400 points: Some Native Americans call their higher power "the Great _____?

answer: the Great Spirit

- For 500 points: People in recovery look for help from a _____?

answer: higher power

- Daily Double: Name five things people can do to restore their spirits?

answer: go to a religious service, walk, meditate, exercise, help someone in need, be with friends, start a personal project, etc.

Self-Care Jeopardy – Social

- For 100 points: Name five things young people can do together to have fun while staying safe.

answer: go to the movies, play basketball, play cards, meet for a soda, go for a walk, …

- For 200 points: It's natural for people to have fun just spending time together? True or False?

answer: True, we are social creatures

- For 300 points: What is it called when your friends urge you to do something with them?

answer: peer pressure

- for 400 points: What qualities do friends show each other?

answer: mutual respect, caring, support, …

- For 500 points: Say the Serenity Pledge from memory?

answer: Give me the serenity to accept the people I cannot change, the courage to change the person I can, and the wisdom to know that person is me!

- Daily Double: What does a good friend do when her friend is getting herself in trouble?

answer: she speaks up or calls 911 if her friend is incapacitated

What I Can Do if I'm Feeling Bored, Lonely or Depressed

Body
1. Brush my teeth, wash my hair, take a shower, wash my clothes
2. Set my alarm to give me a full night's sleep
3. Walk, jog, pump iron, ride a bicycle
4. Play tennis, volleyball, softball, basketball, soccer

Mind
1. Sing, play an instrument, listen to CDs and MP3s, go to a concert
2. Read a book, magazine, newspaper, go to the library
3. Play cards, play a board game, play chess
4. Do my homework, study for a test

Feelings
1. Use paint, ink, chalk, and clay
2. Talk on the phone, online chat, send an email
3. Write in a journal, write in my diary
4. Discuss what's bothering me with someone I trust

Spirit
1. Walk in the country, climb, hike, sit beside a creek
2. Go to church, synagogue, temple or mosque
3. Pray, meditate, sit in a quiet garden
4. Clean up a neighbor's yard, visit a sick friend or relative, help someone with homework, volunteer in a hospital

Social / Being a Kid
1. Join my friends outside
2. Go to the mall with my friends
3. Join a group that champions a good cause
4. Introduce myself to the new kid at school

Goals / Hopes
1. Talk to my school counselor, visit colleges and study their catalogues
2. Go with my parent to 'Bring a child to work day', talk to adults about their work, take an internship
3. Work hard in school, do all my homework, do extra-credit assignments
4. Discuss my future with my parents, my teachers, my school counselors, my pastor or priest

Resolving Conflict Without Violence

<u>By myself or with a safe person</u>:

Who am I having a conflict with? What's it about? Are there any hidden parts of the conflict? What is my role in it?

<u>Approach the person with whom you are having the conflict</u>:

Ask if this is a good time to go over your differences. If not, see if you can arrange a better time. Tell the person your side of the conflict and how you feel about it. Use "I" statements rather than "You" statements to keep tension low. Ask the other person to give his or her side of the conflict. ("How do you see it, and how do you feel about it?") Pay attention and don't interrupt. When the other person is done, summarize and restate what you have heard him or her say, "If I heard you right, this is what you said … Did I get that right?"

<u>Try to work it out</u>:

Tell the other person what you would like to see happen and then ask him or her what he/she would like to see happen. Try to find common ground (what you agree on) and come to a compromise, if possible. If no compromise is possible at this time, agree to disagree and ask if you can talk about it again when you both have had some time to think about what the other has said.

Let's Stop Bullying!

Bullying is Wrong! Nobody has the right to hurt other people by hitting them calling them names, or spreading rumors about them. Bullies justify their actions by saying that it is the victim's fault for being different. They may pick on someone who is tall or small, or fat or thin, or who wears glasses or has red hair, or has a different accent, or another religion, or is shy or clever, or good looking, or disabled, etc. Any excuse will do, and if there is no real reason, then bullies invent one!

It is not your fault! If you are being bullied, it usually has very little to do with you - bullies are unhappy with something in their lives, and hurt others to relieve their own pain. It is the bully's behavior that must change, not yours.

Bullying is about power and control! If a bully can belittle or intimidate you, he/she can control your behavior. This gives the bully a sense of power and control. Once they have control over someone, bullies do not like to have their authority over someone challenged.

Adults can be bullies, too! Bullying is wrong, whatever the age of the person who is doing the bullying. Adults can bully children in many different ways. If an adult is doing something to you, or trying to make you do something you do not think is right, it might be bullying. Talk to someone about what is going on; it will help you know if the adult's behavior is bullying or just normal discipline.

If this is happening at school, you can talk to your parents. If this is happening at home you can talk to a trusted teacher.

Do something! Doing nothing may result in someone getting seriously upset or hurt. That could be you, or the bully might find a new victim. If his/her behavior is not challenged, he/she is not likely to stop.

Do not keep it a secret! The only way to stop bullying is to talk openly about it.

What can you do?

- Talk to someone you can trust - a teacher, parent, older friend or relative.

- Be persistent. If the first person you talk to ignores you, don't give up; speak to someone else.

- Write down everything the bully does or says to you; also, try to write how it makes you feel. Be very careful to write down only things that actually happened. When you find someone you can trust and who is helpful, discuss what you wrote with him or her.

Fill the blanks with things that promote what is in the flower petal.

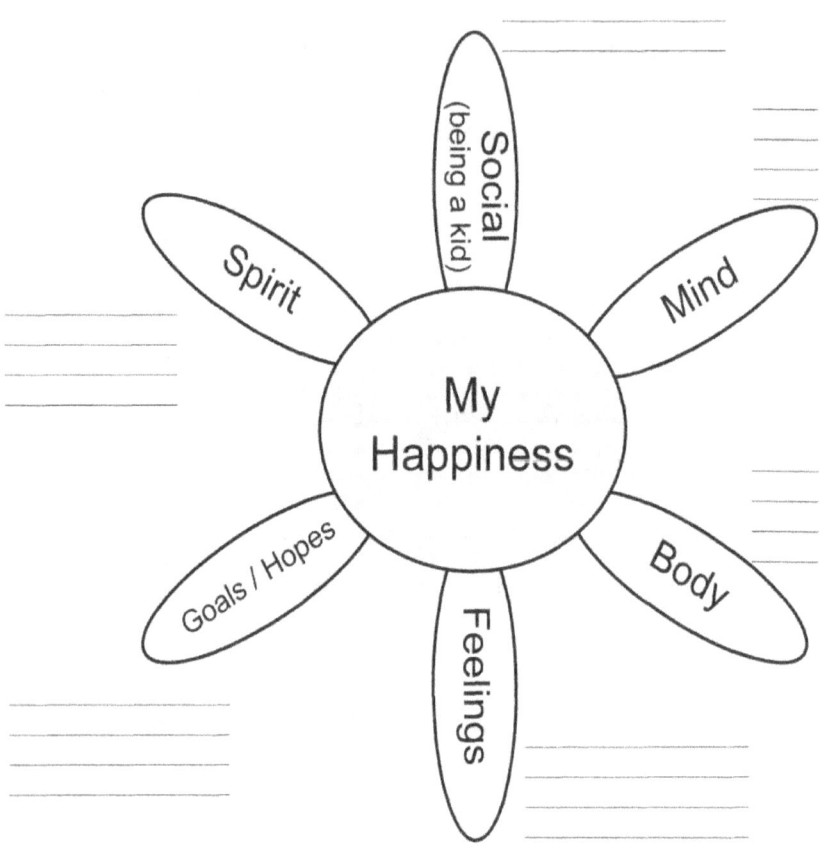

Signs of an Abuser
(for teens and adults)

- Pushes for quick Involvement.   Comes on strong, claiming "I've never felt loved like this by anyone." Pressures you for an exclusive commitment almost immediately.
- Jealous.   Extremely Possessive.   Calls constantly or visits unexpectedly.   Prevents you from going to work because "you might meet someone".   Checks the mileage on your car.
- Controlling.   Interrogates you intensely (especially when you are late) about where you were and who you talked to.   Keeps all the money.   Insists you ask permission to go anywhere or do anything.
- Unrealistic expectations.   Expects you to be the perfect mate and meet his or her every need.
- Isolation.   Tries to cut you off from your family and friends. Accuses people who support you of "causing trouble".   May deprive you of your telephone or car, or try to prevent you from holding a job.
- Blames others for his/her problems or mistakes.   It's always someone else's fault if something goes wrong.
- Makes other responsible for his/her feelings.   Says, "You make me angry" instead of "I am angry" or "you're hurting me by not doing what I tell you".
- Hypersensitive.   Is easily insulted, claiming hurt feelings when he/she is really mad.   Rants about the injustice of things that are just part of life.
- Cruelty to animals or children.   Kills or punishes

animals brutally.   May expect children to do things far beyond their ability (whips or yells at a 3-year-old for wetting a diaper).   Punishes abusively.   May tease or pinch a child until it cries.   (Sixty five percent of abusers who beat their partner will also abuse children.)

- "Playful" use of force during sex.   Enjoys throwing you down or holding you down against your will during sex. Finds the idea of rape exciting.
- Verbally abusive.   Constantly criticizes you or says blatantly cruel things.   Degrades you, curses you, calls you ugly names.   This may involve sleep deprivation, waking you with relentless verbal abuse.
- Rigid gender roles.   Expects you to serve, obey, remain at home.
- Sudden mood swings.   Switches from sweet to violent in minutes.
- Past battering.   Admits to hitting you or another mate in the past but insists the person "made" him/her do it.
- Threats of violence.   Says things like, "I'll break your neck" or "I'll kill you" then dismisses it with "Everybody talks that way" or "I really didn't mean it".

Concluding Thoughts

Growing up in a rather dysfunctional family, I would have found much of this information very useful as a child, even if I had had to read it alone without any adult help. Later, as my wife and I experienced addiction in our own family, the information here would have been of tremendous help to us. The various content was generally available in the facility where our loved one was being treated, but it was not made available to us at the time. When I did become aware of the existence of the materials, I found them to be somewhat unorganized and inconsistent in content from topic to topic. I decided then I would collect and assemble all the information I could find into an organized and consistent whole that I felt would be easier for me to use. That effort was the genesis of what is now this book.

Early on during treatment it was very difficult for me to transition away from a position of "How can I save my loved one's life?" I thought any focus on my own recovery was terribly selfish when another life was so clearly at stake. Eventually I was able to let go of my fear and engage the process that works, that is, self care, along with a full understanding of this disease and the effects it was having on our family. This book contains materials that many people developed, and the underlying approach of the clinic where it was used was for professionals to lead groups of unrelated people through a program very similar to this.

It seems to me that approach is a bottleneck in getting valuable information out to the people who need it, because only small numbers of families have been taking advantage of it and because the information was not being directed at all to the family members of addicts in treatment. I wanted to provide a tool for the community at large, which individual families could use to improve their parenting skills and that families of addicts in treatment would have access to, as well. So, I have reassembled and reconstructed those principles here into a program/package for parents to use in educating their children on a healthy approach to living and growing, whether or not addiction is involved. Of course, when addiction is involved, this book will be even more valuable.   It is important to state, that in cases of addiction in need of treatment, this book is not sufficient. It is to be used only in conjunction with, and supplemental to, the kind of essential primary care and treatment that is offered by the clinics and hospitals that specialize in addiction treatment.

It is my hope that everyone threatened by this disease as well as all the involved family members receive the help and support they need, at the time it is needed. And may that prove sufficient in every single case. I also hope the contents of this book will help others, not impacted by addiction, increase their own family's health and happiness, to the benefit of both parents and the children they are raising.

Thanks to all of you for your support of healthy families.

This book is available from amazon.com in either soft cover or eBook format (with different cover pictures).

www.ingramcontent.com/pod-product-compliance
Lightning Source LLC
Chambersburg PA
CBHW070630290526
45790CB00001B/72